Neur

Essentials: A
Practical Guide

$<$

less

$>$

greater

Neurocritical Care Essentials: A Practical Guide

Mypinder S. Sekhon, MD
Staff Intensivist and Clinical Instructor
Vancouver General Hospital
Division of Critical Care Medicine, Department of Medicine
University of British Columbia
Vancouver, BC, Canada

Donald E. Griesdale, MD, MPH
Staff Intensivist and Assistant Professor
Vancouver General Hospital
Division of Critical Care Medicine, Department of Anesthesiology
Pharmacology and Therapeutics
University of British Columbia
Vancouver, BC, Canada

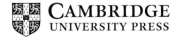

CAMBRIDGE UNIVERSITY PRESS

CAMBRIDGE
UNIVERSITY PRESS

University Printing House, Cambridge CB2 8BS, United Kingdom

Cambridge University Press is part of the University of Cambridge.

It furthers the University's mission by disseminating knowledge in the pursuit of education, learning and research at the highest international levels of excellence.

www.cambridge.org
Information on this title: www.cambridge.org/9781107476257

© Mypinder S. Sekhon and Donald E. Griesdale 2015

First published 2015

Printed in the United Kingdom by Bell and Bain Ltd

A catalog record for this publication is available from the British Library

Library of Congress Cataloging in Publication data
Neurocritical care essentials : a practical guide / [edited by] Mypinder S. Sekhon, Donald E. Griesdale.
    p.   ; cm.
Includes bibliographical references and index.
ISBN 978-1-107-47625-7 (paperback)
I. Sekhon, Mypinder S., 1983–, editor.   II. Griesdale, Donald E., editor.
[DNLM: 1. Central Nervous System – injuries.   2. Central Nervous System Diseases.
3. Critical Care – methods. WL 301]
RC347
616.8–dc23

2014043442

ISBN 978-1-107-47625-7 Paperback

....

Contents

Contributors

William R. Henderson MD FRCPC
Assistant Professor
Division of Critical Care Medicine
Vancouver General Hospital, and
Department of Medicine
University of British Columbia
Vancouver, BC, Canada

Manraj Heran MD FRCPC
Associate Professor
Division of Neuroradiology
Vancouver General Hospital, and
Department of Radiology
Faculty of Medicine
University of British Columbia
Vancouver, BC, Canada

Indeep S. Sekhon MD
Internal Medicine Resident
Department of Medicine
University of British Columbia
Vancouver, BC, Canada

Foreword 1

As our knowledge of the neurosciences continues to expand, so does our ability to diagnose and treat neurological and neurosurgical disorders. The complexity of these cases necessitates critical care, evidenced by the evolution of neuro-critical care units around the world. In recent years, the requirement of neuro-critical care units has been underlined by the improved outcomes of patients admitted to them. In establishing these units, the concept of neurocritical care as a recognized subspecialty of critical care medicine has been realized.

There are many attractions to the subspecialty; the breadth and complexity of the clinical problems that present are both interesting and intellectually challenging. The ability to use advanced technology, whether it be state-of-the-art imaging or neuromonitoring techniques to help clinical decision making, and combining this with the practical diversity of the interventions available to us is both stimulating and rewarding. However, one of the greatest privileges of being part of this small clinical subspecialty is to meet and learn from fellow neurointensivists from around the world. I have been fortunate to work recently with Drs Sekhon and Griesdale, who are not only exemplary clinicians but also dedicated teachers of the specialty. It is therefore not surprising that they have produced this excellent handbook which will be an immensely useful resource not only for healthcare professionals who look after patients within neurocritical care but also for those who look after such patients in non-specialist units.

It is not uncommon to observe our residents (and sometimes attending staff) scratching their heads while on the unit, trying to resolve problems in a timely and appropriate manner. This book will help them with decision making while on service as well as contribute to further understanding of the subject. The chapters are well organized and laid out in a way that makes them easily readable either in depth or for quick reference, so I am sure it will prove a popular resource.

As our subspecialty comes of age, it is reassuring to know that we have such dedicated faculty as are the authors of this book, and that they will train the next generation of neurointensivists to a high standard. The future of neurocritical care is in safe hands.

Professor Arun K. Gupta
Neurocritical Care Unit
Addenbrooke's Hospital
University of Cambridge

Foreword 2

Clinicians who are newly exposed to neurointensive care are burdened with a novel conceptual framework of physiology, pathophysiology and management.

This huge collection of new facts can overwhelm attempts to understand the integrated whole of clinical practice in neurointensive care. While there are many high-quality textbooks on the topic which contain detailed information, these often assume an initial basic framework of knowledge, which may be incomplete (or sometimes absent!).

This handbook provides new entrants to neurointensive care with a useful broad perspective on clinical practice in the subspeciality. The text is both informative and accessible, and will provide an excellent resource for the clinician who wishes to rapidly access key clinical facts, or acquire a foundation to support a wider and more detailed exploration of neurointensive care.

Professor David K. Menon
Neurocritical Care Unit
Addenbrooke's Hospital
University of Cambridge

Acknowledgments

We would like to thank Professor David Menon and Professor Arun Gupta from the Neurocritical Care Unit, Addenbrooke's Hospital, University of Cambridge for providing invaluable guidance and editing suggestions during the production of our book. We would also like to thank our colleagues in the Vancouver General Hospital intensive care unit for their mentorship.

We would like to acknowledge Ms. Alyssa Claire Shook, RN, St. Paul's Hospital, University of British Columbia, for her assistance with formatting and organization of the text.

Finally, we would like to thank our respective families for their support during the production of this text. Their encouragement was invaluable and improved the quality of work.

Mypinder S. Sekhon and
Donald E. Griesdale

Abbreviations

Ab	Antibody
ABC	Airway, breathing, circulation
ABG	Arterial blood gas
ACA	Anterior cerebral artery
ACE	Angiotensin converting enzyme
ACEI	Angiotensin converting enzyme inhibitor
ADC	Apparent diffusion coefficient
ADEM	Acute disseminated encephalomyelitis
ADH	Antidiuretic hormone
AED	Antiepileptic drug
AFB	Acid-fast bacilli
AKI	Acute kidney injury
ALS	Amyotrophic lateral sclerosis
ANA	Antinuclear antibody
ANCA	Antineutrophil cytoplasmic antibody
ANP	Atrial naturetic peptide
ARB	Angiotensin receptor blocker
ARDS	Acute respiratory distress syndrome
ARR	Absolute risk reduction
ARV	Antiretroviral
ARVD	Arrythmogenic right ventricular dysplasia
ASA	Acetylsalicyclic acid
ASA	Anterior spinal artery
ASIA	American Spinal Injury Association
AT	Antithrombin
ATP	Adenosine triphosphate
ATIII	Antithrombin III
AVM	Arteriovenous malformation
BG	Basal ganglia
BG	Blood glucose
BID	Twice daily
BNP	Brain naturetic peptide
BP	Blood pressure
BUN	Blood urea nitrogen
CAD	Coronary artery disease
CaO_2	Arterial oxygen content
CBC	Complete blood count
CBF	Cerebral blood flow

$C_{Br}DO_2$	Cerebral oxygen delivery
CBV	Cerebral blood volume
CCP	Anticyclic citrullinated peptide
CE	Cerebellar encephalitis
CG	Cryoglobulinemia
CI	Contraindication
CIDP	Chronic inflammatory demyelinating polyneuropathy
CK	Creatinine kinase
$CMRO_2$	Cerebral metabolic oxygen uptake
CMV	Cytomegalovirus
CN	Cranial nerves
CNS	Central nervous system
CO_2	Carbon dioxide
COPD	Chronic obstructive pulmonary disease
CPAP	Continuous positive airway pressure
CPP	Cerebral perfusion pressure
CS	Churg–Strauss
CSF	Cerebrospinal fluid
CSW	Cerebral salt wasting
CT	Computed tomography
CTA	Computed tomography angiogram
CVA	Cerebrovascular accident
CvO_2	Cerebral venous oxygen content
CVR	Cerebrovascular resistance
DDAVP	Arginine vasopressin
DE	Diencephalon encephalitis
DI	Diabetes insipidus
DIP	Distal interphalangeal
DKA	Diabetic ketoacidosis
DM	Diabetes mellitus
DVT	Deep vein thrombosis
DWI	Diffusion-weighted imaging
EBV	Ebstein–Barr virus
EDH	Epidural hematoma
EEG	Electroencephalogram
EMG	Electromyography
ENA	Extractable nuclear antibody
EOM	Extraocular movements
ETT	Endotracheal tube
EVD	External ventricular drain
FiO_2	Fractional inspired oxygen
GABA	Gamma-aminobutyric acid
GAD	Gadolinium

GBS	Guillain–Barré syndrome
GCA	Giant cell arteritis
GCS	Glasgow Coma Scale
GI	Gastrointestinal
GN	Glomerulonephritis
Hb	Hemoglobin
HCO^{3-}	Bicarbonate
HELLP	Hemolysis elevated liver enzymes low platelet count
Hep B	Hepatitis B
Hg	Mercury
HHV-6	Human herpes virus 6
HIT	Heparin-induced thrombocytopenia
HIV	Human immunodeficiency virus
HOB	Head of bed
HOCM	Hypertrophic obstructive cardiomyopathy
HONK	Hyperglycemic hyperosmolar non-ketotic coma
HRT	Hormone replacement therapy
HSP	Henoch–Schönlein purpura
HSV	Herpes simplex virus
HTN	Hypertension
IA	Intra-arterial
ICA	Internal carotid artery
ICD	Implantable cardioverter defibrillator
ICH	Intracerebral hemorrhage
ICP	Intracranial pressure
ICU	Intensive care unit
IM	Intramuscular
INH	Isoniazid
INR	International normalized ratio
IP	Interphalangeal
IV	Intravenous
IVH	Intraventricular hemorrhage
IVIG	Intravenous immunoglobulin
LCMV	Lymphocytic choriomeningitis virus
LE	Limbic encephalitis
LMWH	Low molecular weight heparin
LOC	Level of consciousness
LP	Lumbar puncture
LV	Left ventricle
MAOI	Monoamine oxidase inhibitor
MAP	Mean arterial pressure
MCA	Middle cerebral artery
MCP	Metacarpal phalangeal

MEP	Maximal expiratory pressure
MI	Myocardial infarction
MIP	Maximal inspiratory pressure
MM	Multiple myeloma
MPA	Microscopic polyangiitis
MRA	Magnetic resonance angiogram
MRI	Magnetic resonance imaging
MS	Multiple sclerosis
MTP	Metatarsal–phalangeal
NMDA	N-methyl D-aspartate
NMO	Neuromyelitis optica
NNT	Number needed to treat
NSAID	Non-steroidal anti-inflammatory drug
NSE	Neuron-specific enolase
O_2	Oxygen
OCP	Oral contraceptive pill
ODS	Osmotic demyelination syndrome
OER	Oxygen extraction ratio
$PaCO_2$	Arterial partial pressure of carbon dioxide
PaO_2	Arterial partial pressure of oxygen
PAN	Polyarteritis nodosa
PbO_2	Brain tissue oxygenation
$P_{br}O_2$	Brain tissue oxygen pressure
PCA	Posterior cerebral artery
PCR	Polymerase chain reaction
pCO_2	Partial pressure of carbon dioxide
PE	Pulmonary embolism
PEA	Pulseless electrical activity
PEEP	Positive end-expiratory pressure
PIP	Proximal interphalangeal
PMN	Polymorphonuclear neutrophil
PNH	Paroxysmal nocturnal hemoglobinuria
PNS	Parasympathetic nervous system
PRx	Pressure reactivity index
PSH	Paroxysmal sympathetic hyperactivity
PTT	Prothrombin time
RA	Rheumatoid arthritis
RASS	Richmond Agitation Sedation Scale
RCMP	Restrictive cardiomyopathy
RCT	Randomized controlled trial
RE	Rhomboencephalitis
RF	Rheumatoid factor
ROSC	Return of spontaneous circulation

RVOT	Right ventricular outflow tachycardia
SAH	Subarachnoid hemorrhage
SaO$_2$	Arterial hemoglobin oxygen saturation
SBP	Systolic blood pressure
SC	Subcutaneous
SCD	Sequential compression devices
SCI	Spinal cord injury
SDH	Subdural hemorrhage
SIADH	Syndrome of inappropriate antidiuretic hormone
SE	Status epilepticus
SE	Striatal encephalitis
SjO$_2$	Jugular venous bulb oxygen saturation
S$_j$O$_2$ER	Jugular venous bulb oxygen saturation extraction ratio
SLE	Systemic lupus erythmatosis
SNRI	Serotonin norepinephrine reuptake inhibitor
SSEP	Somatosensory evoked potential
SSRI	Selective serotonin reuptake inhibitor
TB	Tuberculosis
TBI	Traumatic brain injury
TCA	Tricyclic antidepressant
TCD	Transcranial Doppler
TIA	Transient ischemic attack
tPA	Tissue plasminogen activator
UE	Upper extremity
UFH	Unfractionated heparin
US	Ultrasound
VC	Vital capacity
VF	Ventricular fibrillation
VGCC	Voltage-gated calcium channel
VGKC	Voltage-gated potassium channel
VKA	Vitamin K antagonists
VT	Ventricular tachycardia
VZV	Varicella zoster virus
WBC	White blood count
WFNS	World Federation of Neurosurgeons Society
WG	Wegener's granulomatosis

Neuroanatomy

Mypinder S. Sekhon and
Donald E. Griesdale

Overall structure and organization

The structure of the central nervous system (CNS) is organized into five distinct parts comprising the cerebrum, diencephalon (thalamus and hypothalamus), brainstem, cerebellum and spinal cord. There is a complex interplay of signals, which are transmitted among each component of the CNS to control consciousness, sensation, motor activity, autonomic nervous function and coordinate speech and movement.

Cerebrum

The cerebrum is composed of the cerebral hemispheres and processes the higher-order functions of the nervous system. It also supplies neuronal connections to nervous system outlets to the voluntary/involuntary muscles and diencephalon, and receives sensory inputs from the peripheral nervous system. The right and left cerebral hemispheres are separated by a central meningeal reflection called the falx cerebri. Posteriorly, the tentorium separates the cerebrum from the intratentorial compartment, which contains the cerebellum and brainstem. Crevices and folds of the cerebrum are referred to as sulci and gyri, respectively. Anatomical boundaries formed by sulci divide the cerebrum into four lobes: frontal, parietal, occipital and temporal. The central sulcus forms the boundary between the frontal and parietal lobes, whereas the Sylvian fissure separates the frontal/parietal lobes from the temporal lobe. The occipital lobe is located posterior to the parietal.

Interhemispheric connections are formed by the corpus callosum, genu and splenium. Deep within the cerebral hemispheres, cavities form the lateral ventricles of the ventricular system, which subsequently drain into the 3rd ventricle.

Importantly, the cerebrum is organized into distinct areas which are responsible for higher-order neurological functions. Nearly 100% of people who are right handed, are left hemisphere dominant, meaning that the language centres are located unilaterally in the left hemisephere. Approximately 75% of

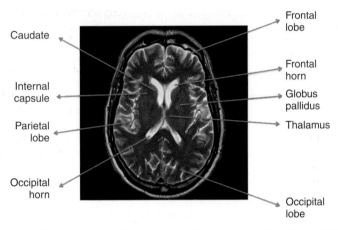

Figure 1.1 MRI axial. An axial MRI slice revealing the appearance of the deep cerebral structures such as the thalami, basal ganglia, internal capsules. Also shown are the frontal and occipital horns of the ventricular system.

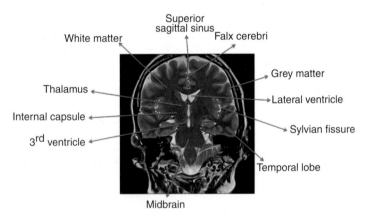

Figure 1.2 MRI coronal. A coronal slice of an MRI demonstrating the appearance of the cerebral hemispheres, cortex and deeper structures such as the thalami and basal ganglia.

left-handed people are also left hemispehere dominant, while the remainder are bilaterally or right-side dominant. The motor area is located immediately anterior to the central sulcus in the major gyrus of the frontal lobe. Alternately, the sensory strip is located in the parietal lobe, in the major gyrus directly opposite to the motor strip. The body's reflection in the sensory and motor strips are organized in the homunculus, which is an anatomical projection in the cerebrum. Centrally, the motor and sensory functions of the feet and lower extremities are located. Moving laterally, the torso, hands and face are anatomically located along the respective gyri.

The speech areas are divided into two distinct regions. Broca's area, which is responsible for expressive speech, is located laterally in the frontal lobe and is bordered by the Sylvian fissure and motor strip. Wernicke's area, which controls receptive speech functions, is located in the temporal and parietal lobes, traversing the Sylvian fissure, and is bordered posteriorly by the occipital lobe.

Diencephalon (thalamus and hypothalamus)

The diencephalon is composed of the deeper structures in the cerebral hemispheres: hypothalamus and thalamus. The thalami, which are located adjacent to the lateral ventricles deep within each cerebral hemisphere serve as a relay centre for sensory input from the body. Sensory neuronal pathways have a connection within the thalami prior to giving rise to the final neuron, which terminates in the sensory cortex of the parietal lobe. The thalamus also has many important connections which regulate the function of the basal ganglia, hypothalamus and cerebellum. Its blood supply arises from the medial and lateral lenticulostriate arteries. It also has a watershed blood supply from the posterior circulation.

The hypothalamus, which is derived from the autonomic nervous system, contains many individual nuclei, each of which has important functions in wakefulness, satiety, hormone production and thermoregulation. Anatomically, it is located superior to the optic chiasm and is connected to the pituitary by the hypophyseal stalk. The hypothalamus is the site of antidiuretic hormone production, which is ultimately stored and released from the posterior pituitary. It is also the site of corticotrophic, thyrotrophic, gonadotrophic and growth hormone releasing hormone production/secretion.

Mesencephalon (brainstem)

The brainstem is composed of three distinct regions: the midbrain, pons and medulla. It is located between the cerebrum and is continuous with the spinal cord caudally. The cerebellum forms its posterior border, making cerebellar pathology a dangerous site of injury if the brainstem is compressed or compromised. The brainstem relays sensory and motor functions between cerebral

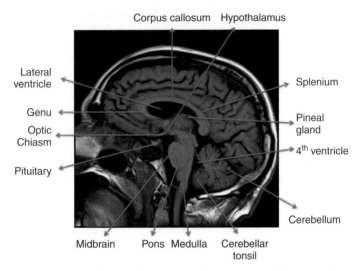

Figure 1.3 MRI sagittal. A sagittal MRI showing the appearance of the corpus callosum, hypothalamus, pituitary and ventricular system. Also shown is the connection between the diencephalon and mesencephalon with the proximity of the cerebellum to brainstem structures in the posterior fossa.

cortex and spinal cord. Additionally, it houses the nuclei of ten of the 12 cranial nerves, which are responsible for important somatic and visceral functions in the body. The reticular activating system is located throughout the brainstem and is principally responsible for wakefulness and arousal. Finally, the respiratory center, which modulates the drive to initiate respiratory effort, is located in the medulla. Complete and irreversible damage to the brainstem and all its functions is determined by clinical examination in the absence of confounders or ancillary tests, and defines brain death.

Cerebellum

The cerebellum is located inferiorly and separated from the occipital lobe by the tentorium. It is divided into hemispheres by a central vermis and is connected to the brainstem via three cerebellar peduncles bilaterally, which carry important neuronal fibres to the peripheral nervous system, cranial nerve nuclei, the diencephalon and basal ganglia. The 4th ventricle and its drainage apertures are located anterior to the cerebellum, making pathology in the cerebellum an important cause of obstructive hydrocephalus if a lesion blocks the ventricular drainage system. The functions of the cerebellum include control of eye movements, speech fluency, coordination of movement and a contribution to proprioception.

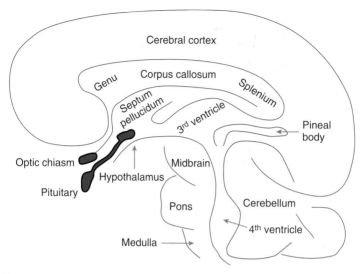

Figure 1.4 Sagittal anatomy of the cerebrum and brainstem. The anatomy of the ventricular system is demonstrated alongside major anatomical structures of the central nervous system. Importantly, the 4th ventricle lies between the cerebellum and brainstem, a narrow area where obstruction to CSF flow can occur, resulting in non-communicating hydrocephalus.

Spinal cord

The spinal cord begins its path caudally from its origin at the medulla and terminates in the conus medullaris at the level of the second or third lumbar vertebral body. The cauda equina extends from the conus as a free standing collection of nerves which exit the spinal column in the lumbosacral region. A cross-section of the spinal cord reveals a butterfly shaped appearance of grey matter which contains cell bodies of motor neurons and important decussating neurons of the spinothalamic tract. In the centre of the cord, the spinal canal is located, which contains cerebral spinal fluid.

The spinal cord is composed of ascending and descending neuronal tracts which carry distinct functions to the peripheral nervous system. Sensory pathways such as the dorsal columns are located posterior to the grey matter and transmit sensations of proprioception, light touch and vibration. The spinothalamic tracts, which carry pain and temperature, have their first-order neuron cross-over in the spinal cord on its ascent in the spinal cord. The major motor tracts, the medial and lateral corticospinal tracts, carry voluntary motor neurons to skeletal muscle. The muscles of the head and neck are carried by the cranial nerves and do not traverse the spinal cord.

Central nervous system blood supply

The brain has dual arterial blood supply from the carotid arteries and vertebrobasilar system. The carotid arteries supply the anterior circulation (frontal, temporal and majority of the parietal lobes). The vertebrobasilar system gives rise to posterior cerebral arteries, which mainly supply the occipital lobes, brainstem and cerebellum.

The right common carotid artery emerges from the brachiocephalic artery and the left common carotid originates directly from the aortic trunk. Both vessels enter the neck and run alongside the internal jugular veins. The common carotid bisects into the internal and external carotid arteries. The external carotid supplies the main extracranial structures of the head and neck. The internal carotid continues its path and eventually enters in the intracranial space via the carotid canal and while running through the cavernous sinus. Once in the intracranial vault, the ICA trisects into the anterior cerebral, middle cerebral and posterior communicating arteries, forming the circle of Willis.

The anterior cerebral artery runs along the base of the frontal lobes and each ACA joins another by the anterior communicating artery. The ACAs supply the medial aspect of the frontal lobe circulation and basal ganglia. The MCA, which is the largest intracerebral artery, runs laterally through the Sylvian fissure and supplies the lateral parts of the frontal and parietal lobes. It also supplies the temporal lobe circulation. Importantly, the lenticulostriate arteries emerge from the MCA proximal to its exit into the Sylvian fissure and supply the deep cerebral structures such as the lateral basal ganglia, internal capsules and thalamus.

The vertebral arteries traverse the spinal column through the intravertebral canals after their origin from the subclavian arteries. Upon exiting the canals, they give rise to the anterior spinal artery, which travels caudally and supplies the anterior two-thirds of the spinal cord. Shortly thereafter, the vertebral arteries join to form the basilar artery at the pons. The posterior inferior and anterior inferior cerebellar arteries originate from the basilar to supply the inferior cerebellum. As the basilar artery travels superiorly, the pontine arteries exit and supply the pons as well as superior midbrain. Finally, the superior cerebellar artery originates from the basilar prior to the basilar artery terminating by giving rise to the posterior cerebral and posterior communicating cerebral arteries in the circle of Willis.

The spinal cord blood supply originates from the vertebral arteries by branches from both forming the anterior spinal artery, which travels caudally to supply the anterior two-thirds of spinal cord. The posterior one-third of the

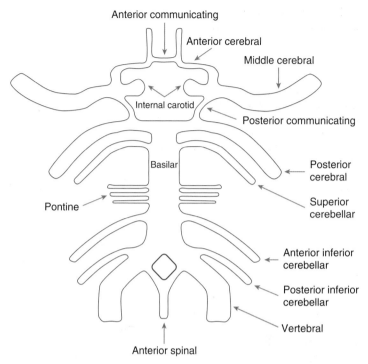

Figure 1.5 Diagram of circle of Willis and cerebral vasculature. The circle of Willis is a confluence of vasculature of the anterior and posterior circulation of the cerebral parenchyma and brainstem. It provides an ability for a source of backup circulatory flow if one source is compromised. The vertebral arteries originate from each subclavian artery and the anterior circulation is provided from the carotid arteries. Branches of the basilar artery supply the entire brainstem and cerebellum.

spinal cord is supplied by the posterior spinal artery, which is supplied by perforators from the intercostal arteries. At the thoracolumbar junction, the artery of Adamkowiez gives rise to the blood supply for the anterior spinal cord. This artery directly originates from the descending aorta.

The venous vasculature of the intracranial space is organized into large venous sinuses, which eventually drain into the internal jugular veins. The superior and inferior sagittal sinus receives venous supply from cortical veins. Interestingly, the superior sagittal sinus also contains arachnoid villi, which absorb CSF into the venous vasculature, the main method of CSF drainage from intracranial space. This large sinus runs along the top of the cerebrum

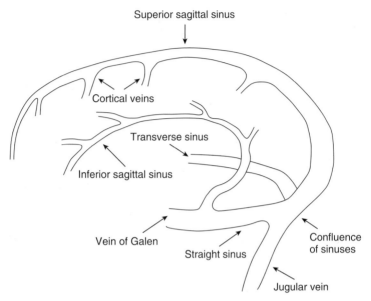

Figure 1.6 Cerebral venous sinus anatomy. Cortical veins drain into both superior and inferior sagittal venous sinuses. The transverse and sigmoid sinuses provide venous drainage from the inferior aspects of the frontal, parietal, occipital and temporal lobes. The vein of Galen drains the deep cerebral structures and forms the straight sinus once joined by the inferior sagittal sinus. Ultimately, all sinuses converge at the confluence of sinuses which leads into the internal jugular veins.

between a fold of dura mater, eventually terminating at the confluence of sinuses located posteriorly. The inferior sagittal sinus drains venous blood from inferior aspects of the frontal and parietal lobes and also terminates in the straight sinus. The transverse sinuses retrieve venous blood from the temporal lobes and run along the tentorium to the confluence of sinuses. The vein of Galen receives venous return from the deep cerebral structures and drains into the straight sinus, which in turn terminates in the confluence of sinuses. From the confluence of sinuses, each internal jugular vein originates and exits the intracranial space via the jugular foramen.

In the cerebral capillaries, the cerebral vasculature exhibits a unique property of a tight barrier function between the intraluminal vascular space and parenchyma. This is termed the "blood–brain barrier" and is formed by numerous tight junctions between the endothelial cells that establish a tightly controlled passage system of substances between the vessels and brain. In states of disease (traumatic brain injury, ischemia, inflammation, infection), the blood–brain barrier can be compromised and leave the brain at risk of edema formation and increased intracranial pressure.

Summary

- The central nervous system is comprised of the cerebrum, diencephalon, brainstem, cerebellum and spinal cord.
- The cerebrum is divided into two hemispheres and controls the high-order functions of the nervous system.
- The brainstem is responsible for transmitting neuronal signals to and from the cerebrum. It also controls wakefulness and contains the respiratory center.
- The cerebellum, located in the posterior fossa, is responsible for balance and cordination.
- The spinal cord is contained within the spinal column and relays messages between the central and peripheral nervous systems.
- The diencephalon is composed of the thalamus and hypothalamus, both of which are situated deep within in the cerebral hemispheres.

Suggested readings

1. Gilman S, Newman S. Manter and Gatz's Essentials of Clinical Neuroanatomy and Neurophysiology, 10th Edition. FA Davis. 2002.

2. Kandel ER, Schwartz JH, Jessell TM. Principles of Neural Science, 4th Edition. Norwalk, CT, Appleton and Lange. 2000.

3. Menon DK. Cardiovascular Physiology. London, BMJ Publishing. 1999.

4. Williams PL. Gray's Anatomy, 38th Edition. Edinburgh, Churchill Livingstone. 1995.

5. Gupta AK, Gelb A. Essentials of Neuroanesthesia and Neurointensive Care, 1st Edition. Elsevier, 2008.

Essential neurophysiology

Mypinder S. Sekhon and
Donald E. Griesdale

Monro–Kellie doctrine

"The cranial cavity is a closed rigid box and that therefore a change in the volume of one of the intracranial compartments can only occur as a result of a compensatory decrease in another compartment(s)."

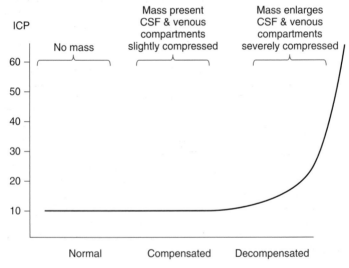

Figure 2.1 Effect of a mass-expanding lesion on intracranial compartment volume and pressure. As the volume of a space occupying lesion increases within the rigid cranium, the CSF and venous vascular compartments gradually decrease to maintain a normal intracranial pressure (ICP). Once these compensatory mechanisms are exhausted, the intracranial pressure rises precipitously and results in herniation. (Adapted from *Textbook of Pediatric Intensive Care, 1996.*)

Table 2.1 Intracranial compartments

Intracranial component	Volume (ml)	%	Compensatory mechanism
Parenchyma	1200	80	None
Vascular	150	10	Increased cerebral venous drainage
Cerebrospinal fluid	150	10	Reabsorption into arachnoid villi CSF drainage into spinal canal

The intracranial pressure and volume curve is an essential physiological concept in the management of brain injury. The Monro-Kellie doctrine states that "the cranial cavity is a closed rigid box and that therefore a change in the volume of one of the intracranial compartments can only occur as a result of a compensatory decrease in another compartment(s)." Thus, the intracranial pressure–volume curve exhibits a sigmoid curve with three distinct zones. In zone 1, the intracranial pressure is low at a normal intracranial volume. In this zone, as the intracranial volume increases, the intracranial pressure remains constant because compensatory mechanisms are able to accommodate for the progressive increase in volume. In zone 2, the intracranial volume continues to expand and compensatory mechanisms become exhausted. This results in a sharp increase in intracranial pressure. In zone 3, the intracranial volume continues to increase but ICP plateaus, which suggests that herniation is occurring.

The RAP index is a linear correlation coefficient between the pulse amplitude of the fundamental component and mean ICP. It is a measure of intracranial compensatory reserve. In the compliant intracranial space, a prominent pulse amplitude exists at a low mean ICP. Therefore, the RAP approximates 0. Once the intracranial compliance deteriorates, the pulse amplitude decreases and approaches the elevated mean ICP. Thus, the RAP approximates +1, a sign of limited compensatory reserve. In zone 3, herniation results in drastically increased ICP with obliteration of the fundamental component and RAP can become negative.

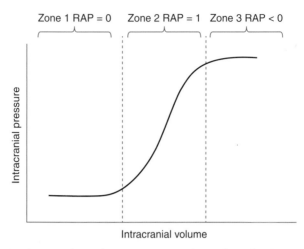

Figure 2.2 Intracranial compliance or pressure–volume relationship. Zone 1 represents good compensatory reserve. Zone 2 has limited compensatory reserve. Zone 3 represents loss of cerebral vascular reactivity and impending cerebral herniation. RAP index = correlation coefficient between pulse amplitude and mean ICP. (Adapted from *Essentials of Neuroanesthesia and Neurointensive Care*, Gupta & Gelb.)

Cerebral oxygen delivery and blood flow

The brain has a high metabolic rate compared with other vital organ systems. It comprises 2% of the body's weight but requires 15–20% of the cardiac output to maintain adequate functioning.

1. The brain requires constant delivery of oxygen and glucose to maintain aerobic metabolism and cellular function as neuronal tissue is devoid of energy stores. In states of starvation, ketones can be utilized. During anaerobic metabolism, there is insufficient production of adenosine triphosphate (ATP) for normal cellular function.
2. Cerebral uptake of oxygen is 3–3.5 ml/100g/min and glucose utilization is 5 mg/100g/min at baseline.
3. Eighty percent of the cerebral blood flow is supplied by carotid arteries and 20% by the verterbrobasilar system. Cerebral blood flow (CBF) parallels cerebral metabolic activity and can vary from 20–80 ml/100g/min. Grey matter is 4× more metabolically active than white matter and prone to global ischemic injury.

Cerebral blood flow regulation is a unique property of the cerebral vasculature-regulating cerebral blood flow to maintain constant delivery of oxygen to the

Table 2.2 Cerebral blood flow regulation

	Category	Clinical state	Response	Clinical application
Intrinsic	Metabolic	Increased	Vasodilate	In normal health, CBF is coupled to cerebral metabolism allowing for matching of cerebral metabolic needs to cerebral delivery of oxygen and glucose
		Decreased	Vasoconstrict	
	Systemic BP (autoregulation)	Hypertension	Vasoconstrict	Maintain steady CBF between MAP 50–150 mmHg. In the setting of chronic HTN, the MAP range of autoregulation is shifted higher
		Hypotension	Vasodilate	
Extrinsic	Blood gases	CO_2 – Hypercarbia	Vasodilate	Vascular response between pCO_2 25–100 mmHg 2–3% change in CBF/mmHg change of pCO_2
		– Hypocarbia	Vasoconstrict	Effect of pCO_2 lost after 24 h due to CSF HCO_3^-
		O_2 – Hyperoxia	Vasoconstrict	Negligible clinical effect
		– Hypoxia	Vasodilate	Vasodilation only if $PaO_2 < 50$ mmHg
	Temperature	Hypothermia	Vasoconstrict	CBF will increase or decrease by 5–7%/degree of temperature (°C)
		Hyperthermia	Vasodilate	
	Blood viscosity	Hyperviscosity	Vasodilate	Optimal Hct 30–35% for CBF
		Hypoviscosity	Vasoconstrict	

cerebral parenchyma. The cerebral vasculature alters the cerebral vascular resistance by vasodilating or vasoconstricting under the influence of many physiological factors.

The cerebral vascular endothelium is principally responsible for maintaining intact cerebral blood flow regulation. In a state of cerebral injury, autoregulation may be impaired, thereby resulting in a near-linear relationship with cerebral perfusion pressure (mean arterial pressure – intracranial pressure) and CBF.

Cerebral autoregulation

Principally, the relationship between the systemic perfusion pressure (mean arterial pressure) and cerebral blood flow describes cerebral autoregulation. In health, CBF is maintained at a constant flow rate over a wide range of mean arterial pressure (MAP), classically described as between 50 and 150 mmHg. Significant variation exists between individuals depending on underlying hypertensive states or concomitant pathology. In states of hypotension, the cerebral vasculature will vasodilate, thereby reducing cerebral vascular resistance and maintaining CBF. Conversely, during hypertension, vasoconstriction occurs and this leads to an increase in cerebral vascular resistance but a constant CBF rate. Below the lower inflection point (MAP < 50 mmHg), the innate ability of the cerebral vasculature is lost and a linear relationship exists between MAP and CBF, potentially leading to cerebral ischemia from inadequate CBF and oxygen delivery. The opposite is true with systemic hypertension (MAP > 150 mmHg), where the linear relationship between MAP and CBF results in pressure passive vasodilation, cerebral hyperemia, vasogenic cerebral edema and risk of hemorrhage.

Carbon dioxide and oxygen

Arterial carbon dioxide tension directly affects CBF in a near-linear relationship over a range of $PaCO_2$ of 25–100 mmHg. Hypercapnia results in cerebral vasodilatation with a CBF increase of 2ml/100g/min of tissue for every 1 mmHg increase in $PaCO_2$. Conversely, hypocapnia results in cerebral vasoconstriction, a manuever that is often used in the management of extreme intracranial hypertension.

Excessive prolonged hypocapnia can result in drastic decreases in CBF and can cause cerebral ischemia, particularly in the injured brain. The effect of hypocapnia-induced cerebral vasoconstriction is a transient phenomenon lasting approximately 18–24 hours due to the reduction in cerebral interstitial bicarbonate over time. This leads to a normalization of cerebral interstitial pH and mitigates the vasoconstriction from therapeutic hyperventilation. A

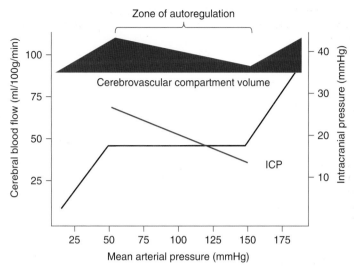

Figure 2.3 Intact autoregulation–normal health. In normal health, the zone of cerebral autoregulation ranges from a mean arterial pressure of 50 mmHg to 150 mmHg. With increasing systemic perfusing pressures, the cerebral arterioles vasoconstrict, which results in a lower cerebrovascular blood volume and, hence, a reduced intracranial pressure within this range. (Adapted from Wartenberg KE, Schmidt JM, Mayer SA. Crit Care Clin 2007 & Neurocrit Care 2004;1:289.)

rebound vasodilation can ensue, which may produce dangerous elevations in ICP in a patient with limited intracranial compliance. Hypoxia results in cerebral vasodilation when PaO_2 falls below 55 mmHg. Alternatively, hyperoxia may result in cerebral vasoconstriction in health but its effect in brain injury is currently unclear.

Temperature

Changes in temperature result in a direct alteration in CBF. Hypothermia leads to a suppression of cerebral metabolic activity ($CMRO_2$). Because of flow metabolic coupling, the reduction in $CMRO_2$ leads to a concomitant fall in CBF. The converse is true with hyperthermia. As a rule, each 1°C change in temperature leads to a 5–7% change in CBF.

Cerebral metabolism

The concept of flow metabolic coupling is a unique property of the brain that allows regulation of blood flow depending on the metabolic activity of the

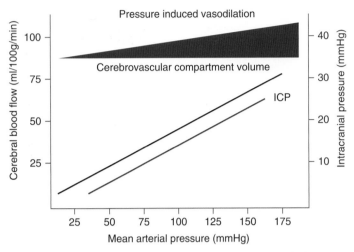

Figure 2.4 Loss of autoregulation–post-cerebral injury. Post-cerebral injury, some patients lose cerebral autoregulation entirely and perfusion of the brain becomes linearly dependent on the systemic perfusing pressure (MAP). In this circumstance, as the systemic perfusing pressure increases, the cerebrovascular compartment volume does as well, ultimately resulting in increased intracranial pressure. The mechanism of increased intracranial pressure can be due to increased cerebral blood volume but also exacerbation of vasogenic cerebral edema from elevated intravascular hydrostatic pressure. (Adapted from Wartenberg KE, Schmidt JM, Mayer SA. Crit Care Clin 2007 & Neurocrit Care 2004;1:289.)

surrounding parenchyma. In short, when cerebral metabolic activity is increased, regional metabolites cause vasodilation and increases CBF. Conversely, when cerebral metabolic activity is reduced by sedation or hypothermia, a reduced level of these metabolites gives rise to an appropriate compensated vasoconstriction that results in a matched reduction in CBF.

Sympathetic nervous system

Stimulation of alpha receptors appears to result in mild cerebral vasoconstriction, albeit to a lesser degree than in the peripheral or splanchnic vasculature. Beta-1 agonism results in regional cerebral vasodilation. The sympathetic nervous system is important in modulation of CBF during autoregulation.

Medications

Various medications have unique effects on CBF and should be used in the appropriate circumstances. Inhalational anesthetics decrease cerebral metabolism

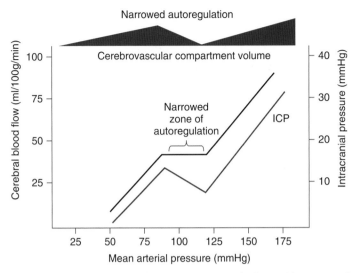

Figure 2.5 Narrowed autoregulation range–post-cerebral injury. The majority of patients who sustain an injury to the brain develop a severely narrowed range of autoregulation over 10–20 mmHg. The majority of these patients have intracranial hypertension and are on the steep portion of the intracranial compliance curve, where small changes in intracranial volume result in large changes in intracranial pressure.

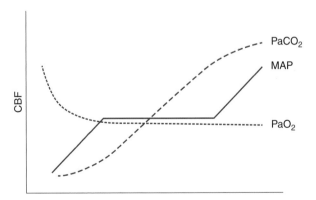

Figure 2.6 Schematic representation of the effect of arterial carbon dioxide and oxygen on cerebral blood flow (CBF). Hypoxia, if extreme ($PaO_2 < 50$ mmHg) results in cerebral vasodilation and a subsequent increase in CBF. Hyperoxia has negligible effects on CBF. Hypocapnia gives rise to cerebral vasoconstriction. Conversely, hypercapnia can produce cerebral vasodilation and increased CBF.

Table 2.3 Important cerebral neurophysiology

$C_{Br}DO_2 = CBF \times CaO_2$
$CaO_2 = (1.34 \times [Hb] \times SaO_2) + (0.003 \times PaO_2)$
$CBF \sim CPP/CVR$
$CPP = MAP - ICP$

$C_{Br}DO_2$ = cerebral oxygen delivery; CBF = cerebral blood flow; CaO_2 = arterial oxygen content of blood; SaO_2 = arterial oxygen saturation; PaO_2 = arterial partial pressure of oxygen; CPP = cerebral perfusion pressure; CVR = cerebral vascular resistance; MAP = mean arterial pressure; ICP = intracranial pressure.

but cause cerebral vasodilation, a state of impaired flow metabolic coupling. Intravenous agents such as propofol, barbiturates and benzodiazepines cause a reduction in cerebral metabolic activity and matched concomitant vasoconstriction, which maintains flow metabolic coupling. Opiates do not to have a significant independent effect on cerebral activity or effects on CBF.

Summary

- Intracranial pressure (ICP) is the pressure placed upon the walls of the lateral ventricles. It is proportional to the sum of the contribution of each intracranial compartment's volume within a fixed intracranial space.
- In the setting of a mass lesion or increased volume of one intracranial compartment, the other two will decrease in volume to maintain a stable ICP.
- The cerebral parenchyma is a metabolically active tissue which relies on aerobic metabolism for energy production and its viability becomes compromised under anaerobic conditions.
- Cerebral blood flow is of paramount importance to maintain adequate oxygen delivery and aerobic metabolism.
- Autoregulation is an inherent quality of the cerebral vasculature that tightly controls cerebral blood flow through the effects of intrinsic and extrinsic factors.
- After sustaining an injury, the cerebral vasculature can lose the ability to autoregulate or the range of autoregulation becomes severely narrowed to 10–15 mmHg.

Suggested readings

1. Paulson OB, Strandgaard S, Edvinsson L. Cerebral autoregulation. Cerebrovasc Brain Metab Rev. 1990 Summer; 2(2): 161–92.

2. Paulson OB, Waldemar G, Schmidt JF, Strandgaard S. Cerebral circulation under normal and pathologic conditions. Am J Cardiol. 1989 Feb 2; 63(6): 2C–5C.

3. Tietjen CS, Hurn PD, Ulatowski JA, Kirsch JR. Treatment modalities for hypertensive patients with intracranial pathology: options and risks. Crit Care Med. 1996 Feb; 24(2): 311–22.

4. Reed G, Devous M. Cerebral blood flow autoregulation and hypertension. Am J Med Sci. 1985 Jan; 289(1): 37–44.

5. Varsos GV, de Riva N, Smielewski P, Pickard JD, Brady KM, Reinhard M, Avolio A, Czosnyka M. Critical closing pressure during intracranial pressure plateau waves. Neurocrit Care. 2013 Mar; 18(3):341–48.

6. Kim DJ, Czosnyka Z, Kasprowicz M, Smieleweski P, Baledent O, Guerguerian AM, Pickard JD, Czosnyka M. Continuous monitoring of the Monro-Kellie doctrine: is it possible? J Neurotrauma. 2012 May; 29(7): 1354–63.

7. Risberg J, Lundberg N, Ingvar DH. Regional cerebral blood volume during acute transient rises of the intracranial pressure (plateau waves). J Neurosurg. 1969 Sep; 31(3): 303–10.

8. Czosnyka M, Citerio G. Brain compliance: the old story with a new 'et cetera'. Intensive Care Med. 2012 Jun; 38(6): 925–7.

9. Gupta AK, Gelb A. Essentials of Neuroanesthesia and Neurointensive Care, 1st Edition. Elsevier, 2008.

Neurological examination

Mypinder S. Sekhon and
Donald E. Griesdale

Chapter 3

The neurological examination consists of four domains: 1. cranial nerve examination 2. motor/reflex/sensory examination 3. cerebellar examination 4. cognitive examination.

Cranial nerve examination

Table 3.1 Cranial nerve functions and examination

Cranial nerve	Function	Examination
I (Olfactory)	Smell	Assess each nostril individually with non-noxious objects
II (Optic)	Visual acuity/fields Colour vision	Snellen chart – acuity Ishihara chart – colour Four-quadrant visual field exam Pupillary light reflex – afferent Accommodation reflex – afferent
III (Oculomotor)	Somatic – EOMs, levator palpebrae Visceral – pupillary constriction	Innervates medial, inferior, superior rectus. Innervates inferior oblique – extorsion Examine EOMs in 6-point position test Pupillary light reflex – efferent Accommodation reflex – efferent
IV (Trochlear)	Superior oblique innervation	Intorsion. Examine each eye by looking "down and in"

Table 3.1 (cont.)

Cranial nerve	Function	Examination
V (Trigeminal)	Facial sensation Masseter/temporalis innervation	V1 – sensory for lateral canthus of eye to vertex. V2 – sensory for corner of mouth to lateral canthus of eye V3 – sensory from edge of mandible to corner of mouth Clench jaw to evaluate muscles of mastication Corneal reflex – afferent
VI (Abducens)	Lateral rectus innervation	Eye abduction. Examine EOMs with 6-point position test
VII (Facial)	Facial muscles innervation Lacrimation/salivation Taste – anterior 2/3 of tongue Sensory of concha/ behind ear	Somatic innervation of frontalis, obicularis oculi, buccinator, obicularis oris and plastysma Taste test of anterior 2/3 of tongue Corneal reflex – efferent Assess mucosa (lacrimation/ salivation)
VIII (Vestibulocochlear)	Hearing Position/balance	Weber and Rhine test Cold calorics Rhomberg test for balance
IX (Glossopharyngeal)	Taste – posterior 1/3 of tongue PNS innervation of pharynx and larynx Innervates pharyngeal muscles	Taste test of posterior 1/3 of tongue Assess swallowing
X (Vagus)	PNS innervation to viscera Gag/cough reflex	Gag/cough reflex Assess uvula Assess swallowing
XI (Accessory)	Innervates trapezius Innervates sternocleidomastoid	Assess shoulder shrug (trapezius) and head turning (sternocleidomastoid)
XII (Hypoglossal)	Tongue movement	Tongue protrusion (tongue will deviate toward side of weakness)

Peripheral motor examination

Table 3.2 Peripheral motor examination and muscle innervation

Peripheral nerve	Myotome	Muscles	Action
Axillary	C5	Deltoids	Shoulder abduction/flexion
Musculocutaneous	C5/C6	Biceps brachii	Elbow flexion/supination
	C5/C6	Coracobrachialis	Elbow flexion/arm adduction
	C5/C6	Brachialis	Elbow flexion
Radial	C6	Supinator	Supination
	C6/C7	Triceps brachii	Elbow extension
	C6/C7	Anconeus	Elbow extension
	C7/C8	Brachioradialis	Pronation/elbow flexion
	C7/C8	Extensor carpi radialis longus/brevis	Wrist extension/hand abduction
	C7/C8	Extensor carpi ulnaris	Wrist extension/hand adduction
	C7/C8	Extensor digitorum	Extend MCP/PIP/DIP (2–5 digits)
	C7/C8	Extensor digiti minimi	Extend MCP/PIP/DIP (5th digit)
	C8/T1	Extensor indicis	Extend MCP/PIP/DIP (index)
	C8/T1	Extensor policis longus/brevis	Thumb extension (IP & MCP)
		Abductor policis longus	Thumb abduction
Median	C6/C7	Flexor carpi radialis	Wrist flexion/hand abduction
	C6/C7	Palmaris longus	Wrist flexion
	C7/C8	Pronator teres	Pronation
	C7/C8	Flexor digitorum superficialis	Flexion of MCP/PIP
	C7/C8	Flexor digitorum profundus	Flexion of MCP/PIP/DIP
	C7/C8	Flexor poilicis longus	Flexion of thumb MCP/IP
	C7/C8	Pronator quadratus	Pronation
	C8/T1	Thenar muscles	Movement of thumb
	C8/T1	Lumbricals to 2/3 digitis	Flexion MCP/extend PIP/DIP

Table 3.2 (cont.)

Peripheral nerve	Myotome	Muscles	Action
Ulnar	C7/C8	Flexor carpi ulnaris	Wrist flexion/hand adduction
	C8/T1	Hypothenar muscles	5th digit adduction/flexion
	C8/T1	Flexor digitorum profundus	Flexion of MCP/PIP/DIP
	C8/T1	Lumbricals to 3/4 digitis	Flexion MCP/extend PIP/DIP
	T1	Interossei	Abduct digits of hand
Femoral branches	L2–L4	Iliopsoas	Hip flexion
Obturator	L2/L3	Gracilis	Hip adduction/knee flexion
	L2–L4	Adductor longus/magnus	Hip adduction
	L3/L4	Obturator externus	Lateral thigh rotation
Femoral	L2/L3	Sartorius	Hip abduction/knee flexion
	L2–L4	Vastus lateralis/medialis/intermedius	Knee extension
	L2–L4	Rectus femoris	Knee extension
Inferior gluteal	L5/S1	Gluetus maximus	Hip extension
Superior gluteal	L5/S1	Gluetus medius	Hip abduction
	L5/S1	Gluetus minimus	Hip abduction
Sciatic	L5–S2	Semitendinosus/semimembranosus	Knee flexion
	L5–S2	Biceps femoris	Knee flexion
Tibial	S1/S2	Lumbricals	Flex MTP/extend PIP, DIP
	S1/S2	Gastrocnemius/soleus	Plantar flexion
	S2/S3	Flexor digitorum longus	Plantar flexion /flexion MTP, IPs
	S2/S3	Flexor digitorum brevis	Flexion MTP, PIP, DIP
	S2/S3	Flexor hallucis longus/brevis	Flexion of great toe MTP/PIP
Common peroneal	L4/L5	Tibialis anterior	Dorsiflexion/inversion
	L5/S1	Extensor digitorum longus	Extend MTP/PIP/DIP of digits 2–5
	L5/S1	Extensor digitorum longus/brevis	Extend great toe

Peripheral reflex examination

Table 3.3 Reflex examination

Reflexes	Nerve	Reflex
Biceps	Musculocutaneous	C5/C6
Brachioradialis	Radial	C6/C7
Triceps	Radial	C7/C8
Knee	Femoral	L3/L4
Ankle	Sciatic/tibial	S1/S2

Peripheral sensory examination

Table 3.4 Peripheral sensory modalities and associated neuroanatomy

Sensory modalities	Fibers	Spinal tract
Light touch	A fibers (myelinated)	Dorsal columns
Proprioception	A fibers (myelinated)	Dorsal columns
Painful stimuli	C fibers (demyelinated)	Spinothalamic
Temperature	C fibers (demyelinated)	Spinothalamic
Vibration	A fibers (myelinated)	Dorsal columns

Table 3.5 Anatomical dermatome landmarks

Dermatome	Location
C5	Shoulder
C6	Lateral aspect of thumb
C7	Lateral aspect of index finger

Table 3.5 (cont.)

Dermatome	Location
C8	Lateral aspect of 5th digit
T1	Medial aspect of forearm
T4	Nipple
T6	Xiphisternum
T10	Umbilicus
T12	Pubic symphysis
L2	Medial aspect of upper thigh
L3	Medial aspect of knee
L4	Medial malleolus
L5	First webspace of foot
S1	Sole of foot
S2/3/4	Perianal space

Table 3.6 Secondary sensory examination and associated tests

Secondary sensory modality	Test
Stereognosis	Recognition of an object in a patient's hand. Inability suggests parietal lobe pathology
Extinction	Simultaneously touching the patient on two different parts of the body. An abnormality in establishing both points of contact suggests parietal lobe pathology
Graphesthesia	Recognition of a printed number or letter on the patient's palm. An abnormality suggests cortical pathology

Cerebellar examination

Table 3.7 Cerebellar examination and associated tests

Test	Clinical information
Nystagmus	Vertical nystagmus can be present with cerebellar pathology
Heel-to-toe	Tests lower limb coordination
Disdiadokinesis	Repetitive tapping of the palmar and dorsal aspect of one hand to the wrist of the other. A test of rapid alternating movements
Finger-to-nose	Tests upper extremity coordination
Gait	Cerebellar pathology produces ataxic, wide-based gait abnormalities
Rhomberg	Positive Rhomberg sign suggests an inability to maintain balance and can be seen with cerebellar pathology

Cognitive examination

Table 3.8 Cognitive examination and associated tests

Test	Clinical information
Level of consciousness	Tested with Glasgow Coma Scale
Orientation	Orientation to time/place/person
Attention	Spelling of WORLD backwards or serial sevens counting down from 100
Visual spatial function	Copying intersecting pentagons as shown on a drawing
Memory	Short-term recall tested with a repetition of three unrelated words (apple, table, penny). Long-term recall tested with recollection of past life events

Neurocritical care scores

Clinical scores

Table 3.9 Grading of motor score

Motor score	Description
0	No movement/flaccid paralysis
1	Flicker movement present/no active movement
2	Voluntary movement but not able to overcome force of gravity
3	Voluntary movement able to overcome gravity but not resistance
4	Voluntary movement able to overcome light resistance
5	Full strength

Table 3.10 Grading of reflexes

Grade	Description
0	No reflex seen
1+	Decreased
2+	Normal
3+	Increased
4+	Clonus

Traumatic brain injury

Table 3.11 Glasgow Coma Score (GCS)

Grade	Glasgow Coma Score
Mild	12–15
Moderate	9–11
Severe	≤ 8

Table 3.12 Glasgow Outcome Scale

1	Dead	Deceased from TBI
2	Vegetative state	Unable to interact with environment, unresponsive
3	Severe disability	Able to follow commands/unable to live independently
4	Moderate disability	Able to live independently, unable to return to school/work
5	Good recovery	Able to return to work/school

Table 3.13 Marshall Score for traumatic brain injury

Category	Description
Diffuse injury I	No visible intracranial pathology on CT
Diffuse injury II	Cisterns are present with midline shift < 5 mm and/or lesion densities present. No high- or mixed-density lesion > 2 5 ml, may include bone fragments or foreign bodies
Diffuse Injury III	Cisterns compressed or absent with midline shift 0–5 mm. No high- or mixed-density lesion > 25 ml
Diffuse injury IV	Midline shift > 5 mm. No high- or mixed-density lesion > 25 ml.
Evacuated mass lesion	Any lesion surgically evacuated
Non-evacuated mass lesion	High- or mixed-density lesion > 25 ml not surgically evacuated

Table 3.14 Rotterdam CT Head Score

Scoring Items	Points	Total score	6-month mortality (%)
Basal cisterns	0 = normal 1 = compressed 2 = absent	1	0%
Midline shift	0 = no shift or ≤ 5 mm 1 = greater than 5 mm	2 3	7% 16%
Epidural mass lesion	0 = absent 1 = present	4 5	26% 53%
Ventricular blood or traumatic SAH	0 = absent 1 = present	6	61%

Subarachnoid hemorrhage

Table 3.15 Clinical classification of subarachnoid hemorrhage

	Hunt & Hess			World Federation of Neurosurgeons	
Grade	Neurodeficit	Survival	Grade	Neurodeficit	GCS
1	None	70	1	Absent	15
2	Headache, neck rigidity	60	2	Absent	13–14
3	Drowsy, mild deficit	50	3	Present	13–14
4	Stuporous, hemiparesis	20	4	Absent or present	8–12
5	Coma, decerebrate	10	5	Absent or present	< 7

Table 3.16 Radiographic classification of subarachnoid hemorrhage

	Modified Fisher Grade			Original Fisher Grade	
Grade	Appearance CT	Vasospasm risk (%)	Grade	Appearance on CT	Vasospasm risk (%)
1	Thin SAH with no IVH	24	1	Focal thin SAH	21
2	Thin SAH with IVH	33	2	Diffuse SAH < 1 mm thick	25
3	Thick SAH with no IVH	33	3	SAH > 1 mm thick	37
4	Thick SAH with IVH	40	4	IVH or intraparenchymal blood	31

IVH = intraventricular hemorrhage, SAH = subarachnoid hemorrhage, CT = computed tomography, Thin SAH < 1 mm thickness, Thick SAH > 1 mm thickness.

Intracranial hemorrhage

Table 3.17 Intracerebral Hemorrhage (ICH) Score

Feature	Points	Total score	30-day mortality (%)
GCS	2 = GCS 3–4 1 = GCS 5–12 0 = GCS 13–15	1	13
ICH volume	1 = > 30 cm³ 0 = < 30 cm³	2	26
IVH	1 = Present 0 = Absent	3	72
Location–infratentorial	1 = Yes 0 = No	4	97
Age	1 = > 80 0 = < 80	5	100

GCS = Glasgow Coma Scale, ICH = intracerebral hemorrhage, IVH = intraventricular hemorrhage.

Sedation score

Table 3.18 Richmond Agitation Sedation Scale

Score	Term	Description
+4	Combative	Violent, danger to self/staff
+3	Very agitated	Aggressive, pulls catheters/lines/tubes
+2	Agitated	Non-purposeful movement, ventilator dyssynchrony
+1	Restless	Anxious
0	Calm	Calm and restful, cooperative
−1	Drowsy	Awakening to voice > 10 seconds with eye contact
−2	Lightly sedated	Awakening to voice < 10 seconds with eye contact
−3	Moderately sedated	Movement to voice, no eye contact
−4	Deeply sedated	Movement/eye opening to physical stimuli only
−5	Unarousable	No response to voice or physical stimuli

Delirium

Table 3.19 The Intensive Care Delirium Screening Checklist

Component	Description	Points
Altered level of consciousness	a. Exaggerated response to normal stimuli (RASS +1 to +4)	1 point
	b. Normal wakefulness	0 points
	c. Response to mild or moderate stimuli	1 point
	d. Response to only intense stimuli	Stop assessment
	e. No response to stimuli	Stop assessment
Inattention	a. Difficulty following commands b. Easily distracted by stimuli c. Difficulty shifting focus	1 point if any present
Disorientation	a. Disorientation to time, place or person	1 point if mistake in any orientation questions
Hallucinations	a. Presence of hallucinations	1 point if hallucinations present
Psychomotor agitation	a. Hyperactivity requiring use of sedative agents or restraints b. Hypoactivity or psychomotor slowing	1 point for either
Inappropriate speech or mood	a. Disorganized, incoherent speech b. Inappropriate mood related to events	1 point if any present
Sleep/wake disturbance	a. Sleeping < 4 h at night b. Waking frequently at night c. Sleeping > 4 h during day	1 point if any pertain to patient
Fluctuating symptoms	a. Fluctuation of any of the above symptoms during preceding 24 h	1 point if any symptoms fluctuant
Total score (1–8)	Score of > 4 has a 99% sensitivity in diagnosing delirium in critically ill patients	

Table 3.20 Full outline of unresponsiveness

Component		Description
Eye response	4	Eyelids open, tracking/blinking to command
	3	Eyelids open but not tracking
	2	Eyelids closed but open to loud voice
	1	Eyelids closed but open to noxious stimuli
	0	Eyelids remain closed despite all stimuli
Motor response	4	Thumbs up, fist or peace sign
	3	Localizing to pain
	2	Flexion response to pain
	1	Extensor response to pain
	0	No response to pain
Brainstem reflexes	4	Pupil and corneal reflexes present
	3	One pupil dilated and fixed
	2	Pupil or corneal reflexes absent
	1	Pupil and corneal reflexes absent
	0	Pupil, corneal and cough reflex absent
Respiration	4	Not intubated, normal respiration
	3	Not intubated, Cheyne–Stokes breathing pattern
	2	Not intubated, irregular breathing pattern
	1	Breathes above ventilator rate
	0	Breathes at ventilator rate or apnea

Approaches to neurocritical care emergencies

Table 3.21 Approach to altered level of consciousness

Approach	Category	Specific etiology
Drugs	Psychotropic meds Sedatives Stimulant withdrawal Anticonvulsants	Typical & atypical anti-psychotics, SSRI/SNRI/MAOI overdose, tricyclic antidepressants, lithium overdose Benzodiazepine, opiates, barbiturates, alcohols Cocaine, amphetamines, LSD, Ecstacy Gabapentin, clobazam, clonazepam, lorazepam, diazepam, phenobarbital
Infection	Systemic infection CNS infection	Septic encephalopathy secondary to organ system infection Meningitis, encephalitis (specifically characterized by altered LOC) Cerebritis, rhomboencephalitis (brainstem infection/inflammation)

Table 3.21 (cont.)

Approach	Category	Specific etiology
Metabolic	Liver	Hepatic encephalopathy, cerebral edema with fulminant liver failure
	Renal	Uremic encephalopathy, metabolic acidemia, electrolyte disturbances
	Electrolyte disturbance	Hypo-/hypernatremia, hypercalcemia, hypophosphatemia
	Hypo-/hyperglycemia	Neuroglycopenia, hyperglycemia (DKA or HONK)
		Acidemia, decompensated hypercapnia
Microvascular	Microangiopathy	Thrombotic thrombocytopenic purpura
		Cholesterol emboli, fat emboli syndrome, vasculitis
		Hypertensive encephalopathy
Structural	Stroke	Ischemic, hemorrhagic, venous thrombosis
	Hemorrhage	Intracerebral, subdural, epidural, subarachnoid
	Malignancy	Primary CNS vs. metastases (lung, breast, melanoma, testicular). Often surrounded by vasogenic edema with mass effect.
	Hydrocephalus	Obstructive vs. non-obstructive
	Infectious	Abscess, cryptoccocoma, tuberculoma
Seizures	Convulsive	Post ictal state after generalized tonic–clonic
	Non-convulsive	Often seen in the critically ill population

Table 3.22 Pertinent history and physical exam in a patient with altered level of consciousness

Category	History	Physical examination
Drugs	Drug intake, empty bottles at scene, previous prescriptions	Elicit physical signs of toxidromes (see Chapter 21)
Infection	Recent fever/illness, symptoms of specific organ dysfunction, travel, sick contacts Symptoms of CNS infection– headache, neck stiffness, photophobia, seizure, altered LOC Immunocompromised	Elicit meningitis signs (Kernig's, Brudzinski's, Hoyne, Asmos signs, neck stiffness, photophobia) Examine each organ system for signs of infection

Table 3.22 (cont.)

Category	History	Physical examination
Metabolic	History of liver/renal impairment, hypoglycemia episodes, electrolyte disturbances Thyroid disturbance	Examine for signs of hepatic failure, uremia, hypo-/hyperthyroid signs
Structural	History of systemic malignancy, stroke, previous intracranial hemorrhage/lesion, concurrent infection, recent head trauma	Evaluate LOC with GCS of FOUR score Brainstem reflexes Focal deficits, upper motor neurons signs Evaluate for papilledema/absent retinal venous pulsations
Seizures	Witnessed seizure, incontinence, tongue biting	Post ictal state, evidence of tongue biting, evaluate for signs of aspiration

Table 3.23 Investigations in a patient with altered level of consciousness

Initial investigations	Utility
Complete blood count	Evaluation for infection, left shift Thrombocytopenia (for TTP)
Electrolytes	Na (hypo- or hypernatremia) Ca (hypercalcemia) Glucose (hypo- or hyperglycemia with DKA/HONK) Bicarbonate (for etiologies of metabolic acidemia) Cl (allows anion gap calculation with bicarbonate)

Table 3.23 (cont.)

Initial investigations	Utility
Urea/creatinine	For uremia, significant renal dysfunction
Liver enzymes and function	For evaluation of hepatic failure
Lumbar puncture	Ensure safety of LP if no contraindications Evaluation for CNS infection/inflammatory condition
Thyroid	Thyroid stimulating hormone
Toxicology screen	For evaluation of illicit substances (opiates, alcohol, benzodiazepines, prior stimulants)
Electrocardiogram	QT prolongation can be seen with psychotropic medication overdose Widened QRS or terminal R wave deflection in aVR with tricyclic antidepressants
Electroencephalogram	Rule out seizures/non-convulsive status epilepticus
Imaging	Computed tomography–non-contrast CT used to rule out major structural causes. Also indicated to rule out contraindications for lumbar puncture Sensitivity is < 50% to detect ischemic stroke within first 24 h of presentation. Require CT angiography to evaluate vasculature. Intracranial lesions (such as malignancies or abscesses) require a CT with contrast

Acute neurological deficit

Table 3.24 Anatomical approach to acute neurological deficit

Approach	Site	Etiology	
Upper Motor	Brain	Vascular	Ischemic or hemorrhagic CVA
		Malignancy	Primary or metastasis
		Infection	Encephalitis, abscess
		Inflammatory	Multiple sclerosis
			Vasculitis, cerebritis
		Hydrocephalus	Obstructive vs. non-obstructive
	Brainstem	Vascular	Hemorrhage/ischemia
		Infection	Rhomboencephalitis
		Inflammation	Ab assoc Rhomboencephalitis
	Spinal cord	Focal lesion	Trauma, hemorrhage, ischemia malignancy, infarction
		Diffuse	Trauma, transverse myelitis ADEM
Lower motor	Anterior horn	Acute	Poliomyelitis
	Peripheral nerve	Demyelinating	Guillain–Barré syndrome
		Axonal	Vaschulitis (mononeuritis multiplex)
			Porphyria
	Neuromuscular junction	Antibody-induced	Myasthenia gravis
			Lambert–Eaton
		Infectious	Botulism
	Muscle	Critical illness	Critical care associated polyneuropathy/ myopathy
		Inflammatory	Dermatomyositis, polymyositis
			Inclusion body myositis
		Endocrine	Hypothyroid, Cushing's
		Toxin/meds	Corticosteroids
			Statins
			Fibrates
			Colchicine
			Cocaine
			Antimalarials

Summary

- The neurological examination consists of assessments of cranial nerves, peripheral motor/sensory/reflexes, cerebellar examination and cognitive evaluation.
- Neurocritical care scores assist in the determination of injury severity and prognosis.
- In TBI, the Glasgow Coma Score establishes injury severity and guides triage.

- CT scores such as the TBI CT Rotterdam Score and Marshall Score correlate with patient outcomes.
- In subarachnoid hemorrhage, scores such as the Fisher/modified Fisher, Hunt & Hess, WFNS Scores all have been shown to correlate with patient prognosis and outcomes.

Suggested readings

1. Kowalski RG, Chang TR, Carhuapoma JR, Tamargo RJ, Naval NS. Withdrawal of technological life support following subarachnoid hemorrhage. Neurocrit Care. 2013. 19(3):269–275.

2. Sung SF, Chen SC, Lin HJ, Chen YW, Tseng MC, Chen CH. Comparison of risk scoring systems in predicting symptomatic intracerebral hemorrhage after intravenous thrombolysis. Stroke. 2013. 44(6):1561–1566.

3. Huang YH, Deng YH, Lee TC, Chen WF. Rotterdam computed tomography score as a prognosticator in head injured patients undergoing decompressive craniectomy. Neurosurgery. 2012. 71(1):80–85.

4. Campbell WW. DeJong's The Neurological Examination. Lippincott Williams & Wilkins. Seventh edition. 2012.

5. Biller J, Gruener G, Brazis P. DeMyer's The Neurologic Examination: A Programmed Text. McGraw-Hill. Sixth edition. 2011.

Neuroimaging

Mypinder S. Sekhon and Manraj Heran

Neuroimaging is a vital aspect of neurocritical care, one which allows a clinician to formulate a diagnosis and also evaluate therapeutic measures. The primary imaging modalities used in critically ill patients with various types of brain injury include computed tomography, angiography and magnetic resonance imaging. Each has its own utility, indications, strengths and weaknesses. A basic understanding of these modalities is essential for clinicians caring for neurocritically ill patients.

Table 4.1 Neurocritical care imaging modalities

Imaging modality	Utility	Strengths	Weaknesses
Non-contrast CT	Evaluation of intracranial hemorrhages, hydrocephalus or acute intracranial process	Readily available Provides sufficient evidence of acute pathology	Unreliable for detecting ischemia. Does not provide detailed imaging of underlying anatomical cerebral parenchyma
Contrast CT	Evaluation of underlying cerebral parenchymal lesion (malignancy, abscess etc.)	Readily available Able to demonstrate underlying intracranial pathology (abscess, malignancy etc)	Contrast administration

Table 4.1 (cont.)

Imaging modality	Utility	Strengths	Weaknesses
CT angiography	Evaluation of cerebral vasculature patency	Readily available Accurate for detecting large-vessel occlusion/ vasospasm/ dissection	Contrast administration No therapeutic capabilities in comparison to conventional angiography
CT perfusion	Evaluation of cerebral blood flow or volume. Use for detecting vasospasm and other conditions of cerebral blood flow compromise	Able to differentiate between established infarcted tissue versus ischemic penumbra which may be rescued with appropriate therapy	Contrast administration High radiation dose
Magnetic resonance imaging	Detailed cerebral anatomical structures	Provides detailed information of underlying cerebral parenchyma and pathology	Not readily available Lengthy examination
MR angiography	Evaluation of cerebral vascular vessel patency and associated vascular pathology	Provides evaluation of underlying cerebral parenchyma and vasculature	Not readily available Contrast administration, although MRI can be done with time of flight sequencing to avoid contrast
Conventional cerebral angiography	Evaluation of cerebral vascular vessel patency and associated vascular pathology	Gold standard for cerebral vascular anatomy and pathological evaluation Therapeutic potential	2% complication rate Requires expertise Contrast administration

Computed tomography

Computed tomography utilizes X-ray beams to penetrate tissues in sequential cuts that produce images at successive levels of anatomical detail in the three-dimensional bodily structure. Tissues have different attenuation depending on:

a. Atomic number of constituent tissues
b. Physical density

Attenuation of a tissue is described as the "attenuation coefficient" and termed "housefield units" on CT.

Contrast-enhanced CT provides greater delineation between normal parenchymal tissue and pathology. Administration of contrast is principally used to identify underlying intracranial lesions such as malignancy, abscesses and other various infectious pathologies of the central nervous system.

Vascular lesions such as arterial aneurysms and arteriovascular malformations require angiography. Detailed examination of the cerebral vessels can be accomplished by computed tomography, magneic resonance imaging or via a conventional angiogram.

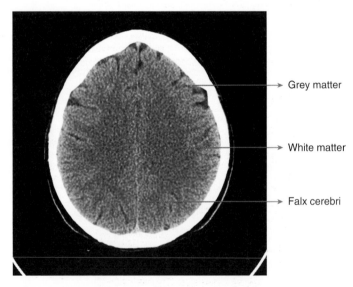

→ Grey matter

→ White matter

→ Falx cerebri

Figure 4.1 Non-contrast CT head. An axial non-contrast CT head revealing the appearance of the motor and sensory cortex. The frontal, parietal and occipital lobes of the cortex are demonstrated with the distinction of grey and white matter. The hemispheres are divided by the falx cerebri.

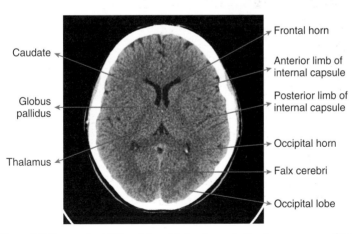

Temporal lobe

Uncus

Basal
cisterns

Midbrain/pons

Posterior
fossa

Figure 4.2 Non-contrast CT head. A lower slice of a head CT demonstrating the appearance of temporal lobes, unci, pons/midbrain and the basal cisterns. This slice is used to identify uncal herniation and basal cistern effacement, which are signs of increased intracranial pressure.

Caudate

Globus
pallidus

Thalamus

Frontal horn

Anterior limb of
internal capsule

Posterior limb of
internal capsule

Occipital horn

Falx cerebri

Occipital lobe

Figure 4.3 Non-contrast CT head. An axial slice demonstrating the appearance of the ventricular system. Also shown is the appearance of the basal ganglia and thalamus, areas which are prone to ischemia in the setting of global hypoxia or cardiac arrest.

Table 4.2 Normal perfusion parameters

Parameter	Grey matter	White matter
Mean transit time	4 seconds	4.8 seconds
Cerebral blood flow	60 ml/100g/min	25 ml/100g/min
Cerebral blood volume	4 ml/100g	2 ml/100g

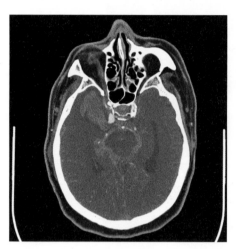

Figure 4.4 CT angiogram. A CT angiogram revealing an aneurysm and associated lobar hemorrhage. The aneurysm orginates from the termination of the internal carotid artery, adjacent to the sella turcica. The associated intraparenchymal hemorrhage extends into the right temporal lobe.

The CT perfusion imaging of the cerebral parenchyma has emerged as a new technique that is able to differentiate between established infarcted tissue and ischemic penumbra which may be "rescue-able" with reperfusion therapy; CT perfusion utilizes three parameters to make the distinction between infarct and penumbra:

a. Mean transit time or time to peak
b. Cerebral blood flow
c. Cerebral blood volume

On CT perfusion, an infarct core is identified by a prolonged mean transit time/time to peak, markedly reduced CBF and CBV. An ischemic penumbra is suggested by prolonged mean transit time/time to peak, moderately reduced CBF and normal or increased CBV because of regional autoregulatory vasodilation from release of local ischemic mediators.

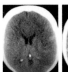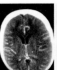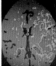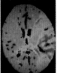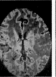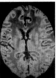

| Non contrast CT | CT Angio | Mean transit time | Time to peak | Cerebral blood flow | Cerebral blood volume |

Figure 4.5 CT perfusion imaging. This series of images demonstrates a non-contrast CT revealing hypoattenuation (indicating ischemia or infarction) in the distribution of the left MCA of a patient with vasospasm post-subarachnoid hemorrhage. The CTA establishes evidence of radiographic vasospasm in the branches of the MCA. There is delayed mean transit time and time to peak in keeping with ischemia or infarct. A marked reduction in the distribution of the left MCA suggests infarct; however, a preserved cerebral blood volume confirms that this patient has a large region of ischemic penumbra. Vasospasm post-subarachnoid hemorrhage with a significant region of penumbra that is "rescue-able" is the final diagnosis.

Magnetic resonance imaging

Magnetic resonance imaging is probably the most versatile neuroimaging tool available. The nucleus of the hydrogen atom (in common with some other elements) is very weakly magnetic, and when placed in a powerful magnetic field, aligns itself longitudinally with the axis of the field. It can be tipped transiently from this equilibrium position into a plane perpendicular to this axis by a radiofrequequency magnetic pulse applied at right angles to the original magnetic field. This transient transverse magnetization is associated with emission of a radiofrequency MR signal that is processed to produce MR images. Removal of the exciting radiofrequency magnetic field results in restoration of equilibrium magnetization, associated with two independent processes:

1. spin–lattice relaxation is the process of recovery of the original longitudinal magnetization, which is characterized by a time constant, T1;
2. spin–spin relaxation is the process by which transverse magnetization decays, and is characterized by a time constant, T2.

Hydrogen nuclei in different tissue environments (e.g., fat, blood, CSF, grey and white matter, pathological tissue) have varying T1 and T2 properties, and also show varying diffusion properties. Different MR imaging protocols (or "sequences") can use these differences to elicit imaging contrasts between tissues.

On T1 sequencing-weighted images, CSF attenuation is dark while white matter exhibits a slightly greater intensity than grey matter. The T1-weighted images reveal more detailed normal anatomical structures. Tissues with short T1 relaxation times appear as bright and conversely, tissues with long relaxation times (cysts, cerebral spinal fluid, edema) appear dark.

Conversely, on T2-weighted images, CSF appears bright and grey matter has a higher signal intensity compared with white matter. On T2-weighted imaging, pathological conditions are shown in greater detail. Tissues with long relaxation times (fluids) appear as bright.

Fluid attenuated inversion recovery (FLAIR) images show the same contrast as T2-weighted images, with the exception that CSF shows low signal, similar to T1 imaging.

Diffusion-weighted imaging uses the microstructural diffusion of water to elicit tissue contrast. Ischemia results in water shift from the extracellular space to the intracellular space (cytotoxic edema). This results in a decrease in the "apparent diffusion coefficient" (ADC) in the extracellular space. The end product is a hyperintensity on DWI, which in the early stages is not accompanied by hyperintensity on T2-weighted images, a combination which is an early signature of ischemia. Later stages of ischemia, and other conditions that disrupt the blood–brain barrier, cause vasogenic edema, which can produce a bright signal on both T2- and diffusion-weighted images. Newer sequences can detect the perturbation in magnetic fields produced by the Fe in hemoglobin, and such "susceptibility-weighted imaging" is exquisitely sensitive to the presence of hemorrhage.

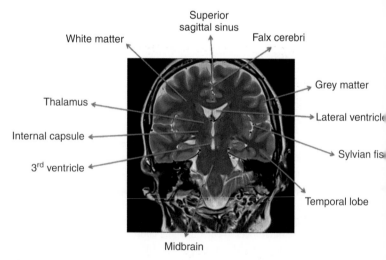

Figure 4.6 MRI coronal. A coronal slice of a MRI demonstrating the appearance of the cerebral hemispheres, cortex and deeper structures such as the thalami and basal ganglia.

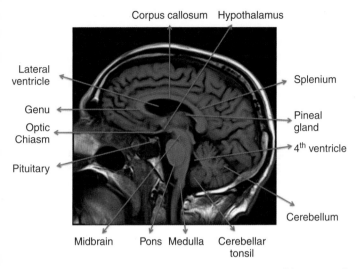

Figure 4.7 MRI saggital. A saggital MRI showing the appearance of the corpus callosum, hypothalamus, pituitary and ventricular system. Also shown is the connection between the diencephalon and mesencephalon with the proximity of the cerebellum to brainstem structures in the posterior fossa.

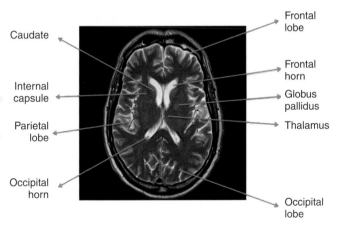

Figure 4.8 MRI axial. An axial MRI slice revealing the appearance of the deep cerebral structures such as the thalami, basal ganglia, internal capsules. Also shown are the frontal and occipital horns of the ventricular system.

Summary

- Neuroimaging is an essential aspect of neurocritical care that guides diagnosis and also therapy.
- Computed tomography has been the mainstay of neuroimaging with the use of non-contrast CT, contrast CT, CT angiography and perfusion.
- Non-contrast CT is predominantly used to evaluate for acute intracranial pathology such as hemorrhage. It has a low sensitivity for detecting acute ischemia.
- Magnetic resonance imaging allows detailed evaluation of the neurological parenchyma and underlying pathology compared to computed tomography.
- T1- and T2- and diffusion-weighted imaging allow for detailed evaluation of the underlying healthy tissue and pathology, respectively.

Suggested readings

1. Symms M, Jager HR, Schmirer K, Yousry TA. A review of structural magnetic resonance imaging. J Neurol Neurosurg Psychiatry. 2004;75:1235–1244.

2. Khan R, Nael K, Erly W. Acute stroke imaging: what clinicians need to know. Am J Med. 2013;126(5):379–386

3. Moseley ME, Liu C, Rodriguez S, Brosnan T. Advances in magnetic resonance neuroimaging. Neurol Clin. 2009;27(1):1–19.

4. Kidwell CS, Wintermark M. Imaging of intracranial haemorrhage. Lancet Neurol. 2008;7(3):256–267.

5. Chalela JA, Kidwell CS, Nentwich LM, et al. Magnetic resonance imaging and computed tomography in emergency assessment of patients with suspected acute stroke: a prospective comparison. Lancet. 2007;369(9558):293–298.

Chapter 5

Neuromonitoring

Mypinder S. Sekhon and
Donald E. Griesdale

Neuromonitoring provides critical diagnostic information on the underlying cerebral pathophysiology and may also afford a therapeutic benefit. Multimodal monitoring provides detailed analysis of cerebral functioning, metabolic activity, cerebral blood flow and cerebral oxygen delivery to help guide management and optimize cerebral functioning.

Modalities

1. Intracranial pressure monitoring devices

1. Normal ICP: 0–10 mmHg, varies with position and age.
2. Intracranial hypertension: ICP > 10–15 mmHg.
3. Treatment threshold: ICP > 20–25 mmHg; however, this may be modified depending on the patient's condition, including other neuromonitoring results.

Table 5.1 Intracranial pressure monitoring device characteristics

Device/location	Accuracy	CSF removal	Hemorrhage rate	Infection rate
Ventriculostomy catheter	Highest accuracy	Yes	0.5%	2–5%
Intraparenchymal	Potential drift in 72–96 h	No	0.1%	0.5–1%
Subdural bolt	Inaccurate	No	< 0.1%	0.1–1%
Epidural bolt	Inaccurate	No	< 0.1%	0.1–1%

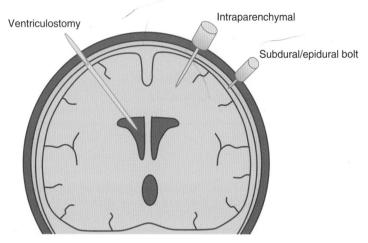

Figure 5.1 Intracranial pressure monitoring device location. The devices available for intracranial pressure monitoring include ventriculostomy catheters, intraparenchymal monitors and subdural bolts. The gold standard of ICP monitoring is the ventriculostomy catheter, which also allows therapeutic cerebrospinal fluid removal capabilities but carries a slightly higher complication rate. Intraparenchymal catheters and subdural bolts yield potentially unreliable readings after 72–96 h due to drift.

Indications for ICP monitoring as per the Brain Trauma Foundation Guidelines

1. TBI with GCS < 8 and abnormal CT scan
2. TBI with GCS < 8 and normal CT with one of the following: age greater than 40 years, episode of hypotension (SBP < 90 mmHg) or posturing

Although the brain trauma foundation guidelines provide reasonable guidance for neuromonitoring indications, they are based on literature from 20–25 years ago. Therefore, careful assessment of the patient and their underlying injury should be considered. The institution of advanced neuromonitoring should be a collaborative approach between the neurosurgery and intensive care foams.

ICP waveform analysis

Compliant cranium

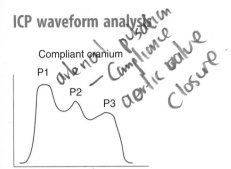

P1

P2

P3

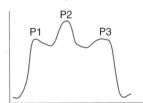

P1 (Percussion wave) = arterial pulsation
P2 (Rebound wave) = intracranial compliance
P3 (Dichrotic wave) = aortic valve closure

Non-compliant cranium

P2

P1   P3

Figure 5.2 ICP waveforms in a compliant and non-compliant cranium. As the cranium transforms into a non-compliant compartment post head injury, the ICP waveform changes from a P1 (percussion wave) dominant wave to a P2 (tidal or rebound wave) dominant wave. P2 is thought to partly reflect the contribution of the cerebral parenchyma, and an accentuation of P2 is often seen following cerebral injury and edema. (Adapted from *J Neurol Neurosurg Psychiatry 2004; 75:813–821.*)

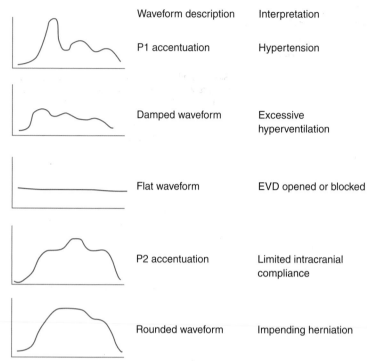

Waveform description	Interpretation
P1 accentuation	Hypertension
Damped waveform	Excessive hyperventilation
Flat waveform	EVD opened or blocked
P2 accentuation	Limited intracranial compliance
Rounded waveform	Impending herniation

Figure 5.3 Variations in ICP waveform and clinical significance. Variations in the ICP waveform can reveal the current state of intracranial compliance and dynamics. Ominous waveforms include a rounded or prominent P2 waveform, which indicate impending herniation and decreased intracranial compliance, respectively. A decrease in amplitude of all three components often occurs after excessive hyperventilation. When an EVD is blocked, kinked or open, a flat waveform ensues. The true ICP is not often relfected with the flat pattern. A prominent P1 is seen during systolic hypertension.

Lundberg waves

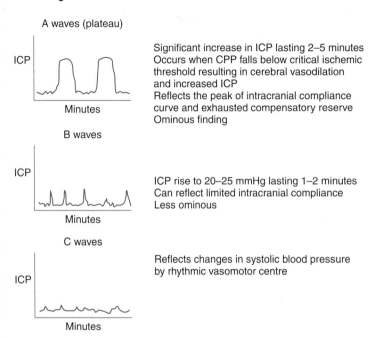

A waves (plateau)

ICP
Minutes

Significant increase in ICP lasting 2–5 minutes
Occurs when CPP falls below critical ischemic threshold resulting in cerebral vasodilation and increased ICP
Reflects the peak of intracranial compliance curve and exhausted compensatory reserve
Ominous finding

B waves

ICP
Minutes

ICP rise to 20–25 mmHg lasting 1–2 minutes
Can reflect limited intracranial compliance
Less ominous

C waves

ICP
Minutes

Reflects changes in systolic blood pressure by rhythmic vasomotor centre

Figure 5.4 Lundberg ICP waves and clinical significance. As the intracranial space crowds and intracranial hypertension ensues, A waves tend to predominate and may indicate impending herniation. The presence of these extreme fluctuations in ICP warrants immediate evaluation and therapy. (Adapted from *J Neurol Neurosurg Psychiatry 2004; 75:813–821.*)

Intracranial pressure monitoring and therapy of controlling increased intracranial pressure are important aspects in various disease processes in neurocritical care. Because the intracranial compartment is a tight rigid box, causes of increased ICP can be attributed to an increase of volume of a particular compartment when the compensatory mechanisms of the remaining two compartments are too exhausted to cope with the increasing volume. The parenchyma can increase in volume as a result of cerebral edema, which in turn has four causes; cytotoxic, vasogenic, hydrocephalic and osmotic.

Cytotoxic edema occurs in the setting of ischemia and cellular energy failure. Insufficient cerebral oxygen delivery results in cellular ion pump failure, intracellular sodium retention and movement of water to the intracellular compartment. This commonly occurs after states of inadequate cerebral oxygen delivery such as cardiac arrest. Vasogenic edema is a result of a breakdown in the normally tight blood–brain barrier. Leakage across the interrupted blood–brain barrier occurs secondary to infection, trauma, ischemia or malignancy. Hydrocephalic edema occurs in the periventricular region in the setting of hydrocephalus. Finally, osmotic cerebral edema occurs with significant swings in the plasma concentrations of osmotically active agents such as sodium and urea. A precipitous decrease in the degree of hypernatremia or uremia can result in cerebral edema due to the retention of organic intracellular osmoles by the neurons.

Table 5.2 Causes of increased intracranial pressure by intracranial compartment

Intracranial compartment	Specific etiology	Pathophysiology
Parenchyma	**Cerebral edema**	
	a. Cytotoxic	Caused by impaired energy-dependent transport of ions, results in intracellular swelling. Occurs after cerebral ischemia.
	b. Vasogenic	Extracellular edema as a result of disruption of the blood–brain barrier. Commonly occurs after a TBI or adjacent to some malignancies.
	c. Hydrocephalic	Occurs in the periventricular region in the setting of hydrocephalus.
	d. Osmotic	Occurs due to shifts in osmotically active molecules between the intra- and extracellular space (i.e., sodium, urea).
Vasculature	**Arterial vasodilation**	
	a. Loss of autoregulation	Causes include a loss of cerebral autoregulation resulting in mild vasodilation in states of increased ICP. In this setting, a small increase in CBV can lead to a large increase in ICP due to limited compensatory mechanisms.
	b. CO_2 and O_2	Other etiologies include hypercarbia and hypoxia.
	Venous obstruction	
	a. Venous thrombosis	Mechanical obstruction to venous outflow caused by reduced intraluminal clots.
	b. Excessive PEEP	Reduced extracranial venous return to the intrathoracic cavity.
	c. HOB down	
	d. Jugular vein obstruction by C-collar or ETT tie	

Table 5.2 (cont.)

Intracranial compartment	Specific etiology	Pathophysiology
Cerebral spinal fluid	**Hydrocephalus**	
	a. Communicating	Decreased CSF absorption from arachnoid villi. Commonly occurs in subarachnoid hemorrhage and cryptococcus meningitis.
	b. Non-communicating	Occurs from an obstruction in the ventricular drainage system proximal to the apertures of Luschka and Magendie.
	Increased CSF production	Occurs with intracranial infection (meningitis or ventriculitis) and choroid plexus tumors.
Other	Malignancy	Primary or secondary tumors. May be associated with per-tumor vasogenic edema or intratumor hemorrhage.
	Hemorrhage	
	a. Epidural	Biconvex appearance on CT.
	b. Subdural	Concavo-convex appearance on CT. Usually results from rupture of bridging cerebral veins.
	c. Intraparenchymal	Most common cause – hypertension.
	Hygroma	Commonly occurs after a TBI associated with a subdural hemorrhage.
	Abscess/subdural empyema	Abscesses can be surrounded by vasogenic edema.

Table 5.3 Clinical and radiographic signs of increased intracranial pressure

Category		Finding	Pathological explanation
Clinical	Symptoms	Headache	Often worse in the morning and exacerbated by straining activities (coughing/sneezing).
		Nausea/emesis	Stimulation to medulla and vagal nerve activation.
	Signs	Papilledema	On fundoscopy, optic disc distension results from CSF diversion into the optic nerve sheath during states of increased ICP. High specificity. Also absent retinal venous pulsations occurs with increased ICP.

Table 5.3 (cont.)

Category		Finding	Pathological explanation
		Cushing's triad	Bradycardia with systemic hypertension and a widened pulse pressure. Low sensitivity. Occurs in response to brainstem ischemia.
		Abducen's nerve palsy	Compression of the sixth nerve at the base of skull.
		Fixed, dilated pupil(s)	With increased ICP in the supratentorial compartment, transtentorial herniation can force the unci of the temporal lobes down through the tentorial notch. This results in compression of the oculomotor nerve nucleus and produces unilateral pupillary dilation and contralateral hemiparesis.
Radiographic	CT	Sulcal effacement	In states of increased ICP, the obliteration of the cerebral sulci can indicate limited space in the intracranial vault.
		Basal cistern effacement	Caudal movement of the intracranial cerebral parenchyma can efface the basal cisterns, a late sign of increased ICP.
		Ventricular collapse	With cerebral edema, the lateral ventricles can become collapsed; a compensatory mechanism of increased CSF drainage to accommodate an increase in volume of the parenchyma or a space occupying lesion.
		Midline shift	Midline shift > 5 mm is significant for possible increased ICP.
		Herniation	Uncal, central and subfalcine herniation can indicate increased ICP. These are also late findings.
	Ultrasound/ MRI	Optic nerve sheath distension	The optic nerve sheath is a continuation of the subarachnoid membrane which surrounds the central nervous system. When ICP increases, CSF is diverted into the optic nerve sheath giving an appearance of a widened sheath on MRI and US. An optic nerve sheath diameter of > 5.5 to 6 mm suggests an ICP > 20.

Troubleshooting ICP monitoring

1. EVDs should be leveled at the level of the foramen of Monro. This is externally approximated at the level of the tragus of the jaw. Not doing so will result in an inaccurate reading. ICP readings with the EVD opened are also not accurate. The EVD must be closed to correctly transduce the ICP.
2. Intraparenchymal monitors can "drift" and yield inaccurate results. If the accuracy of the ICP is in question, the following measures can be undertaken:
   a. Check the ICP waveform to ensure P1/P2/P3 morphology exists.
   b. Check the accuracy of the probe by noting changes in the ICP with maneuvers such as abdominal compression, jugular compression or positioning the patient in the supine position.
      If the ICP increases then the probe is likely functioning. Only conduct these maneuvers if it is safe for the patient (i.e., no increased ICP at baseline).
   c. If an EVD is also in situ, transduce it and compare the ICP readings from the EVD vs. parenchymal probe. A difference of no greater than 2 mmHg should exist.

2. Pressure reactivity index (PRx)

a. PRx is a correlation coefficient between the MAP and ICP.
b. It aims to establish the optimal cerebral perfusion pressure in a patient with cerebral injury at which the injured brain is still autoregulating to provide optimal oxygen delivery.
c. After an injury to the brain, autoregulation can be impaired and a near-linear relationship between CPP and CBF can result. In most patients, this relationship is not completely linear as there is a narrowed window of autoregulation over 10–15 mmHg and PRx attempts to establish this "optimal CPP."

The PRx varies between +1 and −1. Negative numbers indicate that the MAP and ICP are varying in opposite directions, a sign of intact autoregulation. The opposite is true for patients who have lost autoregulation.

In *normal* autoregulation

1. Increased MAP → cerebral vasoconstriction → reduced CBF → decreased ICP.
2. Decreased MAP → cerebral vasodilation → increased CBF → increased ICP.

In either case, both of MAP and ICP vary in *opposite* directions. Therefore, their correlation coefficient (PRx) is negative, indicating intact autoregulation, which provides optimal homogenous cerebral oxygen delivery.

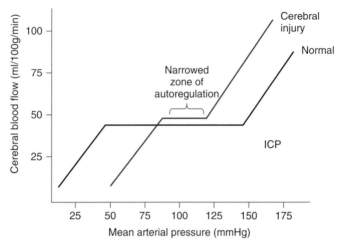

Figure 5.5 Zone of narrowed autoregulation post cerebral injury. Post cerebral injury, the zone of autoregulation in the critically ill traumatic brain injury patient becomes markedly narrowed. The exact range of autoregulation can vary on the type of cerebral injury and underlying co-morbidities, such as systemic hypertension, in each patient. (Adapted from *Anesth & Anal 2008; 107:979–988.*)

In *dysfunctional* autoregulation:

1. Increased MAP → no vascular regulation → increased CBF → increased intracranial vascular volume → increased ICP
2. Decreased MAP → no vascular regulation → decreased CBF → decreased intracranial vascular volume → decreased ICP

In these scenarios, both the MAP and ICP vary in the *same* direction. Therefore, their correlation coefficient (PRx) is positive, indicating dysfunctional autoregulation.

The aim of PRx is to find an optimal CPP at which the PRx is the most negative over a wide range of CPP, thereby establishing the "optimal CPP" in the injured brain. Thereafter the goal is to maintain the actual CPP within proximity of the "optimal CPP" as identified by PRx.

Additionally, monitoring PRx can warn of an impending catastrophic increase in ICP. If the PRx suddenly becomes positive with all other conditions unchanged, this may indicate an impending critical loss in intracranial compliance and should prompt immediate investigation and action.

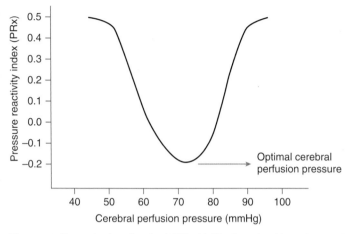

Figure 5.6 Determination of optimal CPP with PRx. By undertaking a therapeutic and diagnostic trial, one can find the "optimal CPP" by gradually adjusting the CPP through manipulation of the cerebral hemodynamics and noting the PRx values over each CPP range. The "optimal CPP" is found once the most negative value of PRx is determined for each CPP. Thereafter, the goal is to maintain the cerebral perfusion pressure within +/− 5 mmHg of the optimal CPP to provide the most effective perfusion and oxygen delivery to the injured brain. (Adapted from *Crit Care Med 2002; 30(4):733–738.*)

3. Brain tissue oxygenation

Brain tissue oxygenation monitors are fiberoptic parenchymal catheters which are placed in the interstitium of the brain and directly measure the pressure of oxygen (PbO_2) in cerebral tissue and serves as a surrogate of cerebral oxygen delivery. A PbO_2 measure of < 10 mmHg is associated with cerebral ischemia and should be avoided. An attempt to maintain the brain oxygenation > 20 mmHg should be made by manipulation of the components of cerebral oxygen delivery.

Brain tissue oxygenation allows focal monitoring of areas of the brain which are at risk of further ischemia and which may not be recognized as undergoing critical ischemia with other more global monitors. It is ideally inserted into the penumbra of the brain injury.

4. Jugular venous oximetry

Analogous to the measurement of a mixed or central venous oxygen saturation in right-sided cardiac circulation, a jugular venous oxygen saturation (SjO_2) measures the venous saturation leaving the brain, thereby providing

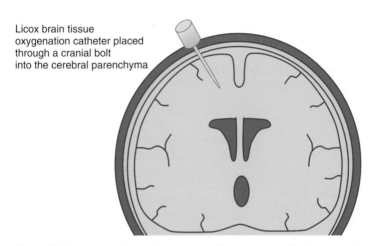

Licox brain tissue
oxygenation catheter placed
through a cranial bolt
into the cerebral parenchyma

Figure 5.7 Positioning of brain tissue oxygenation monitoring. The Licox probe is placed into the cerebral parenchymal through a burr hole and in situ dual-lumen catheter. The Licox probe provides immediate monitoring of the brain oxygen partial pressure within the cerebral parenchyma, which serves as a surrogate for cerebral oxygen delivery. A brain tissue oxygen pressure of < 10 mmHg correlates to cerebral ischemia and adverse patient outcome.

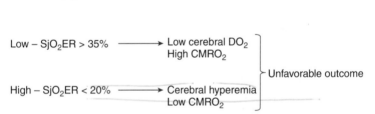

Normal – SjO_2ER 20–35% ⟶ Favorable outcome

Low – SjO_2ER > 35% ⟶ Low cerebral DO_2
High $CMRO_2$

High – SjO_2ER < 20% ⟶ Cerebral hyperemia
Low $CMRO_2$

Unfavorable outcome

Figure 5.8 Jugular venous oximetry and clinical outcome. Maintaining a normal cerebral oxygen extraction is associated with a favourable outcome, while an excessive high or low jugular venous extraction may portend an unfavourable outcome in patients with severe TBI.

information on the balance between cerebral oxygen delivery ($C_{Br}DO_2$) and the cerebral metabolic rate of oxygen utilization ($CMRO_2$).

The goal of TBI management is to minimize secondary ischemic injury and provide adequate cerebral oxygen delivery to at risk, damaged neuronal tissue.

The SjO_2 is a global measure of the balance between oxygen delivery and utilization.

Interpretation:

1. Low SjO_2 = Low $C_{Br}DO_2$ or high $CMRO_2$
2. High SjO_2 = High $C_{Br}DO_2$ (luxury perfusion) or low $CMRO_2$

○ Low SjO_2 ~ High OER

   ✕ SjO_2 55% ~ OER 45%

○ High SjO_2 ~ Low OER

   ✕ SjO_2 85% ~ OER 15%

$$OER = \frac{SaO_2 - SjO_2}{SaO_2}$$

Figure 5.9 Calculation of SjO_2 extraction. The SjO_2 extraction is calculated by analyzing the differences in arterial and jugular venous oxygen saturation. This provides an estimate of the balance of cerebral oxygen delivery and utilization.

$$CMRO_2 = CBF \times (CaO_2 - CvO_2) \qquad C_{Br}DO_2 = CBF \times O_2 \text{ content}$$

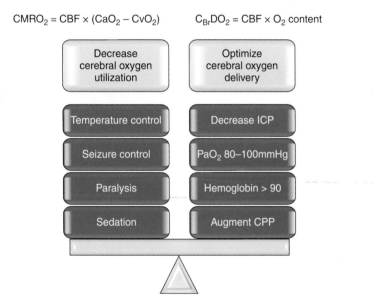

Decrease cerebral oxygen utilization	Optimize cerebral oxygen delivery
Temperature control	Decrease ICP
Seizure control	PaO_2 80–100mmHg
Paralysis	Hemoglobin > 90
Sedation	Augment CPP

Figure 5.10 Approach to the management of TBI with SjO_2. Optimizing cerebral oxygen delivery and minimizing excessive cerebral oxygen utilization is paramount in the management of a severe TBI patient with the use of jugular venous oxygenation saturation monitoring.

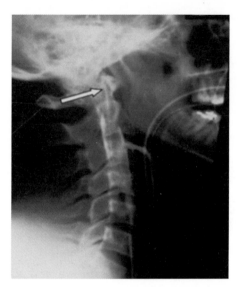

Figure 5.11 Jugular venous bulb catheter placement. The jugular venous catheter should be placed at the level of the mastoid process (white arrow). Sampling should occur over 2 minutes with a gradual aspiration to avoid contamination from the venous drainage of the face.

Placement of catheter:

Ultrasound may be used to assess the size of both jugular veins. The right internal jugular vein is dominant in 65% of patients. The catheter should sit in the jugular bulb, which is located at the level of the mastoid process on lateral cervical spine X-ray.

5. Microdialysis

This technique entails a catheter being placed within the brain interstitium (using the same bolt as the brain tissue oxygenation catheter). Microdialysis catheters have a semipermeable membrane which allows an isotonic fluid to equilibrate with molecular composition of the interstitium, indirectly reflecting intracellular metabolism.

During states of deficient cerebral oxygen delivery, neurons undergo anaerobic metabolism to generate ATP, thereby producing high amounts of lactate. When the interstitium contains elevated lactate/pyruvate ratios, the concentrations of the molecules equilibrate with the isotonic microdialysate and reflect a metabolic crisis when analyzed. Adjustments must be made to augment cerebral oxygen delivery or decrease cerebral metabolism to ensure neurons are not undergoing insufficient energy production and ultimately cell death.

Microdialysis catheter

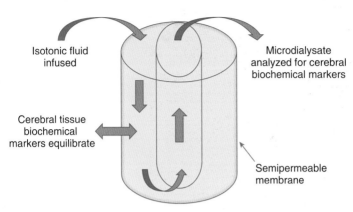

Figure 5.12 Microdialysis mechanism of action. An isotonic fluid is infused into the microdialysis catheter and subsequently the molecular composition of the fluid is analyzed once it returns from the exit port. Due to the semipermeable nature of the catheter's outer walls, molecules within the brain interstitium equilibrate with the microdialysate fluid and then the molecular composition is analyzed. (Adapted from *BJA 2006; 97:18–25.*)

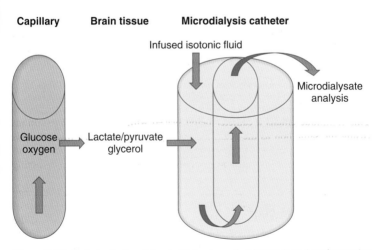

Figure 5.13 Analysis of microdialysate. Molecules such as lactate (a marker of anaerobic metabolism and cerebral ischemia) and glycerol (marker of neuron cell death) can be analyzed in the microdialysate to assess the adequacy of cerebral oxygen delivery and oxygen utilization. (Adapted from *BJA 2006; 97:18–25.*)

Table 5.4 Frequency of seizures and status epilepticus in neurocritically ill patients

Condition	Seizures (%)	Status epilepticus (%)
Ischemic stroke	5	1–10
Subarachnoid hemorrhage	5–15	10–15
Traumatic brain injury	10–30	5–20
Intracranial hemorrhage	20–40	10–30

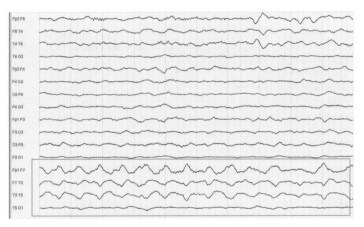

Figure 5.14 Electroencephalogram revealing a subclinical seizure (focal) with slowing over the left lateral/temporal region. In critically ill patients, the majority of seizures are subclinical and the presence of convulsions cannot be relied upon routinely to rule in or out seizures. EEG is required to definitely evaluate for seizures.

6. Continuous EEG

Continuous electroencephalogram monitoring provides a functional assessment of the electrical activity within the brain. It can be helpful in the diagnosis of seizures and their management in the ICU.

The incidence of seizures in the neurocritically ill patients is significant, ranging from 5–50% of patients depending on the underlying condition.

Additionally, the majority of seizures in the ICU are non-convulsive in nature, making the absence of convulsions unreliable in ruling out the diagnosis of seizures or status epilepticus. Additionally, seizures are often transient and can be missed on a brief screening EEG.

7. Transcranial Doppler

Transcranial Doppler (TCD) utilizes a range-gated pulsed Doppler ultrasound beam with a frequency of 2 MHz to assess cerebral blood flow in the major cerebral arteries. The ultrasound beam penetrates the skull in established "windows" and reflects off of erythrocytes. The "Doppler shift" signal is the difference between the transmitted and received signals. The Doppler shift can be expressed as :

$$\text{Doppler Shift} = V \times Ft \times 2 \times cos\theta/C$$

where V = velocity, Ft = frequency, $cos\theta$ is the correction factor for the angle of insonation and C = speed of sound in tissue.

The windows amendable to viewing the intracranial arteries are the temporal (middle cerebral and anterior cerebral arteries), orbital (anterior cerebral arteries), occipital (vertebrobasilar and posterior cerebral arteries). The TCD allows measurement of cerebral vascular reactivity, autoregulation, intracranial pressure and cerebral flood flow. It can be used in subarachnoid hemorrhage, traumatic brain injury and in states of intracranial hypertension. It has also been used intraoperatively in cardiac surgery and carotid endarectomy to assess cerebral flood flow.

Summary

- Multimodal neuromonitoring is the use of several monitoring devices to assess markers of cerebral oxygen delivery, utilization and cerebral activity.
- Invasive intracranial pressure monitoring can warn of dangerous rises in ICP and also assist in calculation of the pressure reactivity index.
- Pressure reactivity index (PRx) provides the determination of the "optimal cerebral perfusion pressure" in each patient and gives insights on intracranial compliance.
- Jugular venous oximetry determines the global cerebral oxygen uptake and utilization balance in the brain.
- Brain tissue oxygenation monitoring is a strategy to target adequate cerebral oxygen delivery to a specific part of the brain or the injured regions (i.e., penumbra).
- Microdialysis assesses the cellular metabolism of neurons after brain injury.
- Continuous EEG gives insights into the incidence of seizures in the neurocritically ill and serves as a therapeutic endpoint to those patients with seizures or status epilepticus.

Suggested readings

1. Wartenberg KE, Schmidt JM, Mayer SA. Multimodality monitoring in neurocritical care. Crit Care Clin. 2007 Jul;23(3):507–38.

2. De Georgia MA, Deogaonkar A. Multimodal monitoring in the neurological intensive care unit. Neurologist. 2005 Jan;11(1):45–54.

3. Bhatia A, Gupta AK. Neuromonitoring in the intensive care unit. II. Cerebral oxygenation monitoring and microdialysis. Intensive Care Med. 2007 Aug;33(8):1322–8.

4. Dunn IF, Ellegala DB, Kim DH, Litvack ZN. Neuromonitoring in neurological critical care. Neurocrit Care. 2006;4(1):83–92.

5. Meixensberger J, Kunze E, Barcsay E, Vaeth A, Roosen K. Clinical cerebral microdialysis: brain metabolism and brain tissue oxygenation after acute brain injury. Neurol Res. 2001 Dec;23(8):801–6.

6. Hillered L, Persson L, Nilsson P, Ronne-Engstrom E, Enblad P. Continuous monitoring of cerebral metabolism in traumatic brain injury: a focus on cerebral microdialysis. Curr Opin Crit Care. 2006 Apr;12(2):112–18.

Chapter

6

Severe traumatic brain injury

Mypinder S. Sekhon and
Donald E. Griesdale

Severe traumatic brain injury (TBI): Blunt or penetrating injury to the brain resulting from trauma and with a presenting Glasgow Coma Scale ≤ 8 in the absence of confounding conditions (e.g., hypothermia, drug intoxication or withdrawal).

Classification

Clinical

Table 6.1 Glasgow Coma Score (GCS)

Grade	Glasgow Coma Score
Mild	12–15
Moderate	9–11
Severe	≤ 8

Currently, TBI is clinically classified by the GCS score. Unfortunately, this approach fails to take into account the underlying diseases/injury in the assessment. For example, a patient with cerebral confusions likely has a different natural history and pathophysiology than another patient with a diffuse axonal injury. Future definitions will hopefully take these nuances into account as our understanding of different types of TBI evolves.

Radiographic/prognosis

Table 6.2 Rotterdam CT Head Score

Scoring items	Points	Total score	6-month mortality (%)
Basal cisterns	0 = normal 1 = compressed 2 = absent	1	0%
Midline shift	0 = no shift or ≤ 5 mm 1 = greater than 5 mm	2 3	7% 16%
Epidural mass lesion	0 = absent 1 = present	4 5	26% 53%
Ventricular blood or traumatic SAH	0 = absent 1 = present	6	61%

Table 6.3 Glasgow Outcome Scale

1	Dead	Deceased from TBI
2	Vegetative state	Unable to interact with environment, unresponsive
3	Severe disability	Able to follow commands/unable to live independently
4	Moderate disability	Able to live independently, unable to return to school/work
5	Good recovery	Able to return to work/school

The Glasgow Outcome Scale has been used as the primary outcome measure in TBI research. Neuro-psychiatric testing is emerging as another useful assessment in clinical studies pertaining to TBI.

Pathophysiology

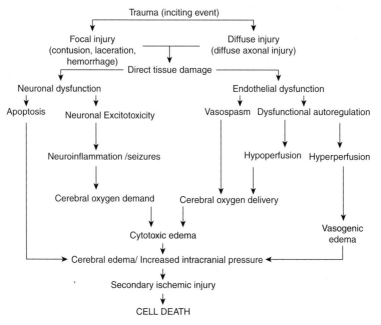

Figure 6.1 Pathophysiology of traumatic brain injury.

Management (severe TBI)

Principles

1. Prehospital care: avoid hypotension SBP < 90 mmHg and hypoxemia PaO_2 < 60 mmHg
2. Transfer to a tertiary trauma centre with neurosurgical and neurocritical care expertise
3. Advanced neuromonitoring (ICP, SjO_2, $PbrO_2$, PRx, cEEG, microdialysis)
4. Prevent secondary ischemic neuronal injury using protocolized care

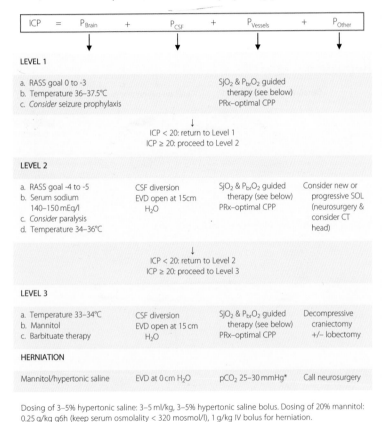

$$ICP = P_{Brain} + P_{CSF} + P_{Vessels} + P_{Other}$$

LEVEL 1

a. RASS goal 0 to -3
b. Temperature 36–37.5°C
c. *Consider* seizure prophylaxis

SjO_2 & $P_{br}O_2$ guided therapy (see below)
PRx–optimal CPP

ICP < 20: return to Level 1
ICP ≥ 20: proceed to Level 2

LEVEL 2

a. RASS goal -4 to -5
b. Serum sodium 140–150 mEq/l
c. *Consider* paralysis
d. Temperature 34–36°C

CSF diversion
EVD open at 15cm H_2O

SjO_2 & $P_{br}O_2$ guided therapy (see below)
PRx–optimal CPP

Consider new or progressive SOL (neurosurgery & consider CT head)

ICP < 20: return to Level 2
ICP ≥ 20: proceed to Level 3

LEVEL 3

a. Temperature 33–34°C
b. Mannitol
c. Barbituate therapy

CSF diversion
EVD open at 15 cm H_2O

SjO_2 & $P_{br}O_2$ guided therapy (see below)
PRx–optimal CPP

Decompressive craniectomy +/– lobectomy

HERNIATION

Mannitol/hypertonic saline

EVD at 0 cm H_2O

pCO_2 25–30 mmHg*

Call neurosurgery

Dosing of 3–5% hypertonic saline: 3–5 ml/kg, 3–5% hypertonic saline bolus. Dosing of 20% mannitol: 0.25 g/kg q6h (keep serum osmolality < 320 mosmol/l), 1 g/kg IV bolus for herniation.
*1 KiloPascal = 7.5 mmHg, SOL = space occupying lesion.

SjO₂ and P_{br}O₂ GUIDED THERAPY

	SjO₂ER < 20% and/or P_{br}O₂ > 50 mmHg	SjO₂ER 20–35% P_{br}O₂ 20–50 mmHg	SjO₂ER > 35% and/or P_{br}O₂ < 20 mmHg
ICP ≤ 20 mmHg	Observe	Observe	a. ↑ CPP to 70–80 mmHg b. Hb ≥ 90 d/l c. pCO₂ 40–45 mmHg
ICP ≥ 20 mmHg	a. Decrease ICP ≤ 20 b. pCO₂ 30–35 mmHg	Decrease ICP ≤ 20	a. Decrease ICP ≤ 20 b. ↑ CPP to 70–80 mmHg c. Hb ≥ 90 d/l

If P_{br}O₂ < 20 mmHg, increase FiO₂ to target PaO₂ > 100 mmHg as temporizing maneuver. Then, adjust CPP or Hb to optimize P_{br}O₂ and reduuce FiO₂ as appropriate.

Herniation syndromes

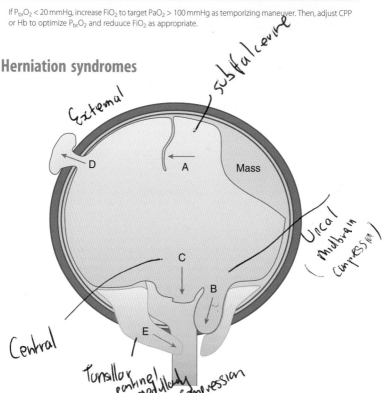

Figure 6.2 Intracranial herniation syndromes. There are five main herniation syndromes (A to D) that can occur with local/diffuse changes in intracranial space and pressure. All can be life threatening with tonsillar, uncal and central herniation causing direct compression of the brainstem. External hernation only tends to occur after a decompressive craniectomy or open skull fracture. Subfalcine hernation can cause contralateral compression of the cerebral hemisphere.

Table 6.4 Clinical significance of herniation syndromes

Letter	Herniation	Cause	Consequence
A	Subfalcine	Unilateral supratentorial mass	Contralateral hemisphere compression
B	Uncal	Unilateral supratentorial mass or increased ICP	Midbrain compression
C	Central	Increased ICP	Midbrain/pons compression
D	External	Open skull fracture, post decompressive craniectomy	Shear hemorrhages at bone/brain interface
E	Tonsillar	Infratentorial mass	Pontine/medulla compression

Table 6.5 Intracranial hemorrhages associated with traumatic brain injury

Category	CT appearance	Notes
Epidural	Convex hyperdensity	Most commonly: middle meningeal artery Associated with skull fracture
Subdural	Concave hyperdensity	Rupture of bridging cerebral veins
Intraparenchymal	Hyperdense collection within parenchyma	Most common sites in trauma include lobar hemorrhages, which are superficially located in contrast to deep cerebral hemorrhage in the basal ganglia in the setting of hypertension
Contusion	Hyper- and hypodensities	Hypodensities represent necrosis of cerebral tissue
Subarachnoid	Hyperdense blood lining the sulci +/− IVH	Traumatic subarachnoid hemorrhage usually focally located and without presence in basal cisterns and ventricles Cause of traumatic SAH is usually a low-pressure venous bleed

External Subfalcine Uncal Tonsillar Central

Figure 6.3 Computed tomography examples of intracranial herniation.

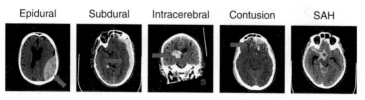

Figure 6.4 Computed tomography of intracerebral hemorrhages associated with TBI.

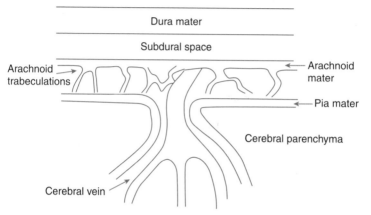

Figure 6.5 **Cross-sectional anatomy of the meningeal layers**. Subdural hemorrhages usually occur following trauma and rupture of the bridging cerebral veins prior to exiting the cerebral parenchyma.

Evidence-based neurocritical care: TBI

Table 6.6 The role of ICP monitoring in severe TBI

Title	A trial of intracranial-pressure monitoring in traumatic brain injury
Author	Chesnut RM.
Summary	RCT of 324 patients with severe TBI admitted to ICU in Bolivia or Ecuador. Patients randomized to intraparenchymal pressure monitor (PM) protocol vs. imaging–clinical examination (ICE). No difference in mortality or GOSE. Concerns of the study include limited generalizability to developed nations' medical systems, increased barbituate use in ICP arm and perhaps that a single ICP < 20 mmHg is not an appropriate target in all brain injuries. This trial may have highlighted the importance of multimodal monitoring to individualize therapy for TBI patients.

Table 6.7 The role of decompression in TBI

Title	Decompressive craniectomy in diffuse traumatic brain injury (DECRA)
Author	Cooper DJ.
Summary	DECRA RCT of 155 patients randomized to bifrontal decompressive craniectomy resulted in lower ICPs but worse clinical outcomes (GOS-E) at 6 months compared to stardard care.

Table 6.8 The role of magnesium infusions in severe TBI

Title	Magnesium sulfate for neuroprotection after traumatic brain injury: a randomised controlled trial
Author	Temkin NR.
Summary	Magnesium infusion resulted in no reduction in composite endpoint (mortality, seizures, functional measures and neuropsychological tests) at 6 months, or mortality in RCT of 499 patients with TBI (GCS ≤ 12). In fact, patients who received a low target (1.00–1.85 mmol/l) had worse outcomes.

Table 6.9 The role of therapeutic hypothermia in severe TBI

Title	Very early hypothermia induction in patients with severe brain injury (the National Acute Brain Injury Study: Hypothermia II): a randomised trial (NABIS: H II)
Author	Clifton GL.
Summary	Conflicting data exist on the possible benefits of therapeutic hypothermia. NABIS: H II was an RCT of early hypothermia of short duration (48 h) in 97 patients with TBI (GCS ≤8); it demonstrated no difference in GOS at 6 months. Trial was stopped for futility. Awaiting results of Eurotherm 3235 trial.

Summary

- Traumatic brain injury classification is stratified based on initial GCS scores in the absence of confounding variables.
- Cerebral edema can occur after TBI and subsequent intracranial hypertension may ensue. The peak of cerebral edema and intracranial hypertension post TBI is typically 3–6 days post injury.

- The pathophysiology of TBI leads to secondary isch which can result in additional cerebral edema and ir
- Multimodal neuromonitoring is used to optimize and prevent secondary ischemic injury to the cere
- In the setting of extreme intracranial hypertensio can ensue.

Suggested readings

1. Vincent JL, Berre J. The medical management of severe traumatic brain injury. Crit Care Med. 2005;331:392–400.

2. Li L, Timofeev I, Czosnyka M, Hutchinson PA. The surgical approach to the management of increased intracranial pressure after traumatic brain injury. Anesthesia Analog. 2010;111(3):736–749.

3. Wright WL. Sodium and fluid management in acute brain injury. Curr Neurol Neurosci Rep. 2012;12:466–473.

4. Rosenfeld JV, Maas AI, Bragge A, Morganti-Kossmann C, Manley GT, Gruen RL. Early management of severe traumatic brain injury. Lancet. 2012;380;1088–1098.

5. Maas AI, Stochetti N, Bullock R. Moderate and severe traumatic brain injury in adults. Lancet Neurol. 2008;7:728–741.

6. Chesnut RM, Temkin N, Carney N, et al. A trial of intracranial-pressure monitoring in traumatic brain injury. N Engl J Med. 2012;367:2471–2481.

7. Cooper DJ, Rosenfeld J V, Murray L, et al. Decompressive craniectomy in diffuse traumatic brain injury. N Engl J Med. 2011;364(16):1493–1502.

8. Temkin NR, Anderson GD, Winn HR, et al. Magnesium sulfate for neuroprotection after traumatic brain injury: a randomised controlled trial. Lancet Neurol. 2007;6(1):29–38.

9. Clifton GL, Valadka A, Zygun D, et al. Very early hypothermia induction in patients with severe brain injury (the National Acute Brain Injury Study: Hypothermia II): a randomised trial. Lancet Neurol. 2011;10(2):131–139.

Subarachnoid hemorrhage

Mypinder S. Sekhon and
Donald E. Griesdale

Intracranial hemorrhage originating in the subarachnoid space may be either aneurysmal or non-aneurysmal in etiology.

Table 7.1 Etiology of subarachnoid hemorrhage

Subarachnoid hemorrhage			
Cause	**Frequency**	**SAH location**	**Clinical pearls**
Aneurysmal	85%		
Anterior cerebral	20%	Diffuse cortical	Higher frequency of
Middle cerebral	20%	Basal cisterns	complications
Posterior cerebral & posterior communicating	15%	Ventricles	Prognosis worse
Anterior communicating	20%		
Other (carotid/basilar)	10%		
Etiology	**Frequency**	**SAH location**	**Clinical pearls**
Non-aneurysmal	15%		
Perimesencephalic	10%	Midbrain	Prognosis excellent
Arterial dissection	5%	Basal cisterns	History of neck trauma, CN deficits
Arteriovenous malformation		Superficial	Family history

Table 7.1 (cont.)

Etiology	Frequency	SAH location	Clinical pearls
Dural arteriovenous fistula		Basal cisterns	Previous history of head trauma/fracture
Septic/mycotic aneurysm		Superficial	Concurrent or previous systemic infection
Cocaine		Variable	Concurrent sympathomimetic toxidrome
Trauma		Variable	Concurrent TBI
Pituitary apoplexy		None	Visual symptoms/signs
Spinal cord vascular lesion		Basal cisterns	History of back pain between shoulders

TBI = traumatic brain injury, SAH = subarachnoid hemorrhage, CN = cranial nerves.
(Adapted from *Brain 2001; 124:249–278.*)

Classification

Table 7.2 Clinical classification of subarachnoid hemorrhage

Hunt & Hess			World Federation of Neurosurgeons		
Grade	Neurodeficit	Survival	Grade	Neurodeficit	GCS
1	None	70	1	Absent	15
2	Headache, neck rigidity	60	2	Absent	13–14
3	Drowsy, mild deficit	50	3	Present	13–14
4	Stuporous, hemiparesis	20	4	Absent or present	8–12
5	Coma, decerebrate	10	5	Absent or present	< 7

Table 7.3 Radiographic classification of subarachnoid hemorrhage

Modified Fisher Grade			Original Fisher Grade		
Grade	Appearance on CT	Vasospasm risk (%)	Grade	Appearance on CT	Vasospasm risk (%)
1	Thin SAH with no IVH	24	1	Focal thin SAH	21
2	Thin SAH with IVH	33	2	Diffuse SAH < 1 mm thick	25
3	Thick SAH with no IVH	33	3	SAH > 1 mm thick	37
4	Thick SAH with IVH	40	4	IVH or intraparenchymal blood	31

IVH = intraventricular hemorrhage, SAH = subarachnoid hemorrhage, CT = computed tomography. Thin SAH < 1 mm thickness, Thick SAH > 1 mm thickness.

Diagnosis

Table 7.4 Diagnostic imaging of subarachnoid hemorrhage

		Test Characteristics	
Diagnostic test	Objective	Sens/Spec (%/%)	Special notes
CT non-contrast	Detection of SAH	90–95/90–95	Decreased sens > 48 h post SAH
Lumbar puncture	Detection of SAH	70–80/95–100	Xanthochromia > 12 h post SAH
CT angiogram	Aneurysm detection	85–98/90–95	Decreased sens for aneurysm < 5 mm

Table 7.4 (cont.)

Diagnostic test	Objective	Test Characteristics	
		Sens/Spec (%/%)	Special notes
MR angiogram	Aneurysm detection	70–90/75–90	Decreased sens for aneurysm < 5 mm
Cerebral angiogram	Aneurysm detection +/– therapeutic	95–100/95–100	Gold standard; 2% complication rate

Cerebrovascular aneurysm

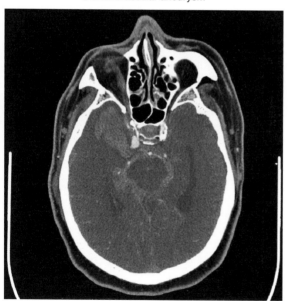

Figure 7.1 CT angiogram demonstrating a cerebral aneurysm located at the origin of the middle cerebral artery. An adjacent lobar hemorrhage is seen. The aneurysm, which is located in proximity to the bifurcation of the internal carotid and middle cerebral artery, is a common location for cerebral vascular aneurysms.

1. New focal neurological deficit
2. Decreased level of consciousness

Rule out structural complications
a) Rebleed (if not secured)
b) Hydrocephalus
c) Vasospasm

Obtain CT angiogram (with CT head) or CT perfusion

If neurological deterioration not explained by CT
head/angiogram / perfusion then pursue EEG to
rule out status epilepticus

Figure 7.2 Approach to neurological deterioration in SAH. It is imperative to rigorously follow the neurological examination in subarachnoid hemorrhage patients and minimize sedation to follow for neurological deterioration. Prompt evaluation with dedicated neuroimaging analyzing for complications such as rebleed, obstructing hydrocephalus and vasospasm should be initiated in the setting of neurological deterioration. If these investigations do not reveal a cause of deterioration, the diagnosis of seizures and status epilepticus should strongly be considered and warrants immediate EEG evaluation.

SAH

Vasospasm

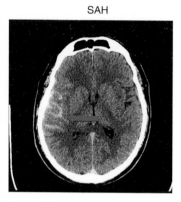
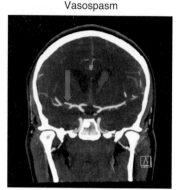

Figure 7.3 Computed tomography subarachnoid and accompanying cerebral vasospasm. Evidence of subarachnoid blood in the basal cisterns suggests an aneurysmal nature of the SAH. The left-hand image reveals an area of vasospasm in the distribution of the middle cerebral artery post aneurysmal SAH. Vasospasm risk starts from day 3–4 post SAH and peaks at day 7–12. The risk gradually dissipates over days 14–28 post aneurysmal SAH.

Post SAH vasospasm

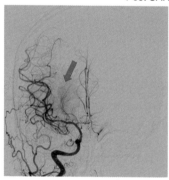
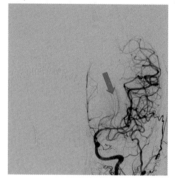

Figure 7.4 Conventional angiogram of a subarachnoid hemorrhage patient with cerebral vasospasm. The tethering of the cerebral vasculature after an SAH indicates radiographic evidence of vasospasm, which can result in cerebral ischemia and infarction.

Monitoring & goals	General ICU care	SAH specific therapy
• SaO$_2$ ≥ 97% • Mean arterial pressure monitoring • Glucose: as per ICU insulin protocol • Hemoglobin ≥ 90 d/l • Serum Na > 135 mEq/l	• DVT prophylaxis – SCDs • GI prophylaxis • Nutrition • HOB 30° • Neurovitals every hour	• Nimodipine 60 mg every 4 hours • Maintain euvolemia • Maintain normal magnesium • Temperature 36–37.5°C

Aneurysmal subarachnoid hemorrhage

Secure aneurysm within 48 h by endovasculcar coiling or microvascular clipping

Unsecured aneurysm
a. SBP < 140 mmHg   b. Tranexamic acid (if delay to coil or clip >72 h)   c. Coagulopathy reversal

Secured aneurysm
a. If coiling or clipping, keep SBP < 140 mmHg unless evidence of acute vasospasm. If vasospasm, MAP goal 90 –140 mmHg 6 hours post clip/coil.

Management of complications

Complication	Management
Vasospasm (moderate to severe)	Initial therapy – induced hypertension Hypertension – MAP goal 90:140 mmHg If concomitant LV dysfunction then: milrinone – 0.125mcg – 0.75mcg/kg/min IV infusion, maintain MAP goal If failed induced hypertension therapy, then consider: intra-arterial angioplasty (for proximal large-vessel vasospasm) intra-arterial vasodilators (nicardipine or milrinone) Reassess efficacy of vasospasm treatment (clinical exam +/− imaging every 24–48 h)
Hydrocephalus	Cerebrospinal fluid diversion External ventricular drain placement (EVD), set at 5–10 cm H$_2$O initially Serial lumbar puncture or lumbar drain if communicating hydrocephalus only

	If EVD in place: leave open at 5–15cm H_2O, notify neurosurgery of failure of EVD to drain Culture CSF if suspicion for ventriculitis and/or every 24–48 h
Na^+ Disorders	Hyponatremia – SIADH vs. cerebral salt wasting Avoid fluid restriction. Use hypertonic saline for correction. Consider fludrocortisone for cerebral salt wasting Hypernatremia Rule out central diabetes insipidus DDAVP 1–2 mcg every 12 h for Na goal of 135–145 if DI
Cardiac	Arrythmias Telemetry, maintain normal electrolytes (especially K^+/Mg^{2+}) Cardiomyopathy Obtain echocardiogram for suspicion of new left ventricular dysfunction Consider inotropes (dobutamine/milrinone) if requiring vasopressor support
Seizures	Obtain EEG if: convulsive seizures persistently/fluctuating/new decreased level of consciousness Management: first-line anticonvulsant – phenytoin 20mg/kg IV load then 5–7mg/kg IV q8h refer to status epilepticus protocol

The following case demonstrates a patient who presented with complete right-sided hemiparesis and expressive/receptive aphasia secondary to severe left MCA vasospasm on day 7 post subarachnoid hemorrhage. The initial non-contrast CT demonstrates an area of hypoattenuation which suggests ischemic/infarcted tissue. The subsequent CTA reveals vasospasm in the distal branches of the MCA. The CT perfusion imaging revealed delayed time to peak, mean transit time, reduced CBF but preserved CBV, indicating a large area of ischemic penumbra as opposed to established infarct. The patient was managed with induced hypertension treatment and repeat imaging demonstrated a marked improvement in the hypoattenuation on non-contrast CT, radiographic vasospasm, time to peak and mean transit time. The CBF returned to normal and CBV increased post treatment. Most importantly, the patient recovered from neurological deficits of receptive and expressive speech as well as right-sided motor function.

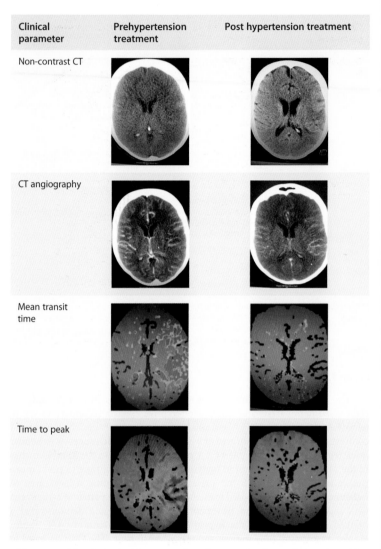

Figure 7.5 CT perfusion imaging pre- and post hypertensive therapy for a patient with post SAH vasospasm.

Clinical parameter	Prehypertension treatment	Post hypertension treatment
Cerebral blood flow		
Cerebral blood volume		
Neurological exam	Expressive and receptive aphasia. Right arm and leg hemiparesis.	Resolution of expressive and receptive aphasia. Full power of right lower extremity. 3/5 motor strength of right upper extremity.

Figure 7.5 (cont.)

Table 7.5 Grading of vasospasm post SAH

	Conventional angiography		CT or MRI angiography
Grade 1	Vasospasm in one vascular axis	None	No vasospasm
Grade 2	Vasospasm in two vascular axes	Mild	< 50% reduction in vessel caliber
Grade 3	Vasospasm in three vascular axes	Moderate	50–75% reduction in vessel caliber
Grade 4	Diffuse or generalized vasospasm	Severe	> 75% reduction in vessel caliber

Evidence-based neurocritical care

Table 7.6 The ISAT trial

Title	International subarachnoid aneurysm trial (ISAT) of neurosurgical clipping versus endovascular coiling in 2143 patients with ruptured intracranial aneurysms: a randomised comparison of effects on survival, dependency, seizures, rebleeding, subgroups, and aneurysm occlusion
Author	Molyneux AJ.
Summary	ISAT RCT of 2143 patients with a hSAH in whom the aneurysm was amenable to either approach demonstrated a lower risk of death or dependence at 1 year in the endovascular coilling (23.5%) vs. surgical clipping (30.9%) (p < 0.001). This benefit persisted up to 7 years. Higher risk of rebleeding in coiling after procedure but offset by higher risk of rebleeding while awaiting surgery. Long-term risk of rebleeding was small in both groups. This study had a highly select group of patients, higher risk of rebleeding in coiling group after procedure was offset by higher risk of rebleeding while awaiting surgery.

Table 7.7 The role of calcium channel blockers in SAH

Title	Calcium antagonists for aneurysmal subarachnoid haemorrhage
Author	Dorhout Mees SM.
Summary	Meta-analysis of RCTs demonstrates that oral nimodipine (calcium antagonist) reduces the risk of poor outcome (16 trials, RR 0.67, 95% CI 0.55 to 0.81) and secondary ischemia (11 trials, RR 0.66, 95% CI 0.59 to 0.75) following aneurysmal SAH.

Summary

- Subarachnoid hemorrhage is classified as either aneurysmal or non-aneurysmal in etiology.
- Severity of an aneurysmal subarachnoid hemorrhage is graded by clinical findings and radiographic features.
- The management of subarachnoid hemorrhage is to prevent the known complications which can occur post SAH and maintain adequate cerebral oxygen delivery.
- Cerebral vasospasm post SAH is a significant cause of mortality and morbidity. The incidence is correlated directly with the severity of grade of the SAH.

Suggested readings

1. van Gijn J, Rinkel GJE. Subarachnoid hemorrhage: diagnosis, causes and management. Brain. 2011;124:249–278.

2. Muroi C, Seule M, Mishima K, Keller E. Novel treatments for vasospasm after subarachnoid hemorrhage. Curr Opin Crit Care. 2012;18:119–126.

3. Conolly S, Rabinstein A, Carhuapoma R, Derdeyn C, et al. Guidelines for the management of aneurysmal subarachnoid hemorrhage: A guideline for healthcare professionals from the American Heart Association/American Stroke Association. Stroke. 2012;43(6):1711–1737.

4. Diringer MN, Bleck TP, Hemphill C, Menon D, et al. Critical care management of patients following aneurysmal subarachnoid hemorrhage: Recommendations from the Neurocritical Care Society's Multidisciplinary Consensus Conference. Neurocrit Care. 2011;15:211–240.

5. Green DM, Burns JD, DeFusco CM. Management of aneurysmal subarachnoid hemorrhage. J Intensive Care Med. 2012;28(6):341–354.

6. Frontera JA, Claassen J, Schmidt JM, Wartenberg KE, Temes R, Connolly ES Jr, MacDonald RL, Mayer SA. Prediction of symptomatic vasospasm after subarachnoid hemorrhage: the modified Fisher scale. Neurosurgery. 2006;59(1):21–27.

7. Fisher CM, Kistler JP, Davis JM. Relation of cerebral vasospasm to subarachnoid hemorrhage visualized by computerized tomographic scanning. Neurosurgery. 1980;6(1):1–9.

8. Lannes M, Teitelbaum J, del Pilar Cortés M, Cardoso M, Angle M. Milrinone and homeostasis to treat cerebral vasospasm associated with subarachnoid hemorrhage: the Montreal Neurological Hospital protocol. Neurocrit Care. 2012 Jun;16(3):354–362.

9. Molyneux AJ, Kerr RSC, Yu L-M, et al. International subarachnoid aneurysm trial (ISAT) of neurosurgical clipping versus endovascular coiling in 2143 patients with ruptured intracranial aneurysms: a randomised comparison of effects on survival, dependency, seizures, rebleeding, subgroups, and aneurysm occlusion. Lancet. 2005;366(9488):809–817.

10. Molyneux AJ, Kerr RSC, Birks J, et al. Risk of recurrent subarachnoid haemorrhage, death, or dependence and standardised mortality ratios after clipping or coiling of an intracranial aneurysm in the International Subarachnoid Aneurysm Trial (ISAT): long-term follow-up. Lancet Neurol. 2009;8(5):427–433.

11. Dorhout Mees SM, Rinkel GJE, Feigin VL, et al. Calcium antagonists for aneurysmal subarachnoid haemorrhage. Cochrane Database Syst Rev 2007;(3):CD000277.

Intracranial hemorrhage

**Mypinder S. Sekhon and
William R. Henderson**

Spontaneous intraparenchymal hemorrhage with or without intraventricular extension.

Etiology

Table 8.1 Approach to etiology of intracerebral hemorrhage

Category	Causes	Notes
Primary	Hypertension	Most commonly located in deep cerebral tissues (i.e., basal ganglia, thalamus, pons, internal capsule)
	Amyloid angiopathy	Typically causes lobar hemorrhages

Secondary	Neoplasm	Malignancies predisposed to hemorrhage
		– Glioblastoma multiforme
		– Metastatic malignancies
		  – Melanoma
		  – Breast
		  – Testicular
		  – Renal cell

	Vascular a. AVM b. Aneurysm c. Angioma	CT or MR angiography required to delineate underlying lesion
	Trauma	Lobar hemorrhages located superficially
	Venous thrombosis	Multiple hemorrhages, often in distribution of major cerebral venous sinus
	Hemorrhagic transformation of ischemic stroke	Associated with surrounding ischemic penumbra
	Drugs – sympathomimetics	Similar location of hypertensive etiology
	Coagulopathy	Usually underlying lesion present

AVM = arteriovenous malformation, CT = computed tomography, MR = magnetic resonance.

Diagnosis

CT scan

The CT scan readily demonstrates acute hemorrhage as a hyperdense signal intensity (see image below). Multifocal hemorrhages at the frontal, temporal or occipital poles suggest a traumatic etiology. Intracranial hemorrhage: CT scan of right frontal intracerebral hemorrhage complicating thrombolysis of an ischemic stroke.

Hematoma volume in cubic centimetres can be approximated by a modified ellipsoid equation: $(A \times B \times C)/2$, where A, B and C represent the longest linear dimensions in centimetres of the hematoma in each orthogonal plane.

Perihematomal edema and displacement of tissue with herniation also can be appreciated.

Iodinated contrast may be injected to increase screening yield for underlying tumor or vascular malformation.

The CT angiography "spot sign" may be used to predict growth of intracerebral hematomas.

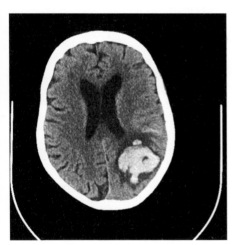

Figure 8.1 Computed tomography of frontotemporal intracerebral hemorrhage. An intracerebral hemorrhage is shown with surrounding cerebral edema and contralateral cerebral hemispheric compression.

Intracerebral hematoma   Presence of spot sign   Expansion of hematoma

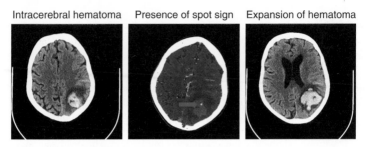

Figure 8.2 Computed tomography of intracerebral hemorrhage with spot sign and expansion. The presence of a spot sign indicates active extravasation of blood during the time of the CT, which predicts interval expansion of the intracerebral hemorrhage. (Adapted from *Neurology* 2010; 75:834.)

Magnetic resonance imaging

Table 8.2 Magnetic resonance imaging stages of intracerebral hemorrhage

Phase	Time	Hemoglobin	T1	T2
Hyperacute	< 24 hours	Oxyhemoglobin (intracellular)	Iso or hypo	Hyper
Acute	1–3 days	Deoxyhemoglobin (intracellular)	Iso or hypo	Hypo
Early subacute	> 3 days	Methemoglobin	Hyper	Hypo
Late subacute	> 7 days	Methemoglobin (extracellular)	Hyper	Hyper
Chronic	> 14 days	Hemosiderin (extracellular)	Iso or hypo	Hypo

Management

Evaluate for secondary cause if location of hemorrhage and history are not compatible with HTN.

Table 8.3 General management principles

Monitoring & goals	General ICU care	Investigations
• SaO$_2$ ≥ 97% • Central venous and arterial catheter • Glucose: 6–10mmol/L	• DVT prophylaxis – SCDs • GI prophylaxis • Nutrition • HOB 30°	• Admission EEG within 48 h • CT head angiogram • CBC, INR/PTT, fibrinogen

Table 8.4 Approach of intracerebral hemorrhage management

Prevent hematoma expansion	Neuroprotection	Surgical therapy
SBP < 140 mmHg Coagulopathy reversal[4] Plts > 100 INR < 1.5 PTT < 40	Temperature 36–37.5°C Na > 140 mEq/l Seizure evaluation (Tx if present) Glucose 6–10 mmol/L ICP/CPP guided therapy	Surgical decompression[1, 2] External ventricular drain[3]

[1] Infratentorial indications: a. > 3 cm b. Brainstem compression c. Hydrocephalus

[2] Supratentorial indications: a. Herniation b. Hydrocephalus.

[3] Indications: a. Hydrocephalus b. ICP monitoring if GCS < 8 or evidence of herniation.

[4] Coagulopathy reversal: a. Coumadin – Octaplex or fresh frozen plasma for immediate reversal. Vitamin K onset ~ 8–12 hours b. Platelet inhibitors – consider platelet transfusion c. Unfractionated heparin – protamine.

Table 8.5 ICP guided therapy in intracranial hemorrhage

LEVEL 1

a. RASS goal 0 to −3   PRx – optimal
b. Temperature 36–37.5°C   CPP

↓

ICP ≥ 20 for > 5 minutes (not stimulated), open EVD and drain CSF, then close EVD
ICP < 20: return to Level 1
ICP ≥ 20: proceed to Level 2

LEVEL 2

a. RASS goal −4 to −5	CSF	PRx –	Consider new or progressive
b. Serum sodium	Diversion	optimal CPP	neurosurgery & consider CT
145–155 mEq/l	EVD at 15		head
c. *Consider* paralysis	cm H_2O		
d. Temperature 35–36°C			

HERNIATION

Osmotherapy	Open EVD	pCO_2	Call neurosurgery
(mannitol & hyperteonic		25–30 mmHg	
saline)			

Prognosis

Table 8.6 Intracerebral Hemorrhage (ICH) Score

Feature	Points	Score	30-day mortality (%)
GCS	2 = GCS 3–4 1 = GCS 5–12 0 = GCS 13–15	1	13
ICH volume	1 = > 30cm^3 0 = < 30 cm^3	2	26
IVH	1 = Present 0 = Absent	3	72
Location – infratentorial	1 = Yes 0 = No	4	97
Age	1 = > 80 0 = < 80	5	100

GCS = Glasgow Coma Scale, ICH = intracerebral hemorrhage, IVH = intraventricular hemorrhage.

Evidence-based neurocritical care

Table 8.7 The INTERACT trial

Title	Rapid blood-pressure lowering in patients with acute intracerebral hemorrhage
Author	Anderson CS.
Summary	INTERACT2 RCT of 2839 patients with spontaneous ICH (GCS med, IQR was 14, 12–15) randomized to SBP < 140 mmHg vs. SBP < 180 mmHg. Although no difference in death or severe disability at 90 days, improved functional outcomes on modified Rankin score (OR 0.87, 95% CI 0.77 to 1.00, p = 0.04) with SBP < 140 mmHg. However, this excluded patients with structural cause, need for surgery or coma.

Table 8.8 The role of activated Factor VII in ICH

Title	Efficacy and safety of recombinant activated factor VII for acute intracerebral hemorrhage
Author	Mayer SM.
Summary	Recombinant activated factor VII (rFVIIa). The RCT of 841 patients with ICH randomized to either placebo, rFVIIa (20 mcg/kg) or rFVIIa (80 mcg/kg). Although receiving rFVIIa at 80 mcg/kg resulted in significant reduction in growth of ICH, there was no difference in severe disability or death at 90 days. Additionally, higher doses of rFVIIa appear to increase the risk of arterial thromboembolic events.

Table 8.9 The role of early surgery in ICH

Title	Early surgery versus initial conservative treatment in patients with spontaneous supratentorial lobar intracerebral haematomas (STICH II): a randomised trial
Author	Mendelow AD.
Summary	Two large RCTs have examined the role of surgery in ICH. STICH randomized 503 patients to early (< 24 h) surgery with medical management. No difference in favourable outcomes at 6 months, although 26% in medical arm crossed over to evacuation. STICH II examined early surgery vs. medical management in superficial lobar ICH of 10–110 ml in 601 patients. Once again, no difference in unfavourable outcome between groups. However, there may be subgroups that benefit: those with poor prognosis or deterioration after presentation.

Summary

- There are numerous causes of an intracerebral hemorrhage, each of which has characteristic clinical and imaging findings.
- The diagnosis of ICH involves determination of hemorrhage with computed tomography and then additional imaging or laboratory invetigations to evaluate for the underlying cause.
- The management of ICH aims to prevent additional hematoma expansion, provide neuroprotection and use surgical techniques, if indicated, to protect the viable cerebral parenchyma.

Suggested Readings

1. Grise EM, Adeoye O. Blood pressure control for acute ischemic and hemorrhagic stroke. Curr Opin Crit Care. 2012;18:12–138.

2. Flower O, Smith M. The acute management of intracerebral hemorrhage. Curr Opin Crit Care. 2011;17:106–114.

3. Nyquist P. Management of acute intracranial and intraventricular hemorrhage. Crit Care Med. 2010;38:946–954.

4. Diringer MN. Intracerebral hemorrhage: pathophysiology and management. Crit Care Med. 1993;21(10):1591–1603.

5. Tatu L, Moulin T. Prognosis and treatment of spontaneous intracerebral hematoma: review of the literature. J Neuroradiol. 2003;30(5):326–331.

6. Steiner T, Bösel J. Options to restrict hematoma expansion after spontaneous intracerebral hemorrhage. Stroke. 2010;41(2):402–409.

7. Qureshi AI, Palesch YY, Martin R, Novitzke J, Cruz-Flores S, Ehtisham A, Ezzeddine MA, Goldstein JN, Hussein HM, Suri MF, Tariq N. Antihypertensive treatment of acute cerebral hemorrhage study investigators. Effect of systolic blood pressure reduction on hematoma expansion, perihematomal edema, and 3-month outcome among patients with intracerebral hemorrhage: results from the antihypertensive treatment of acute cerebral hemorrhage study. Arch Neurol. 2010;67(5):570–576.

8. Qureshi AI, Harris-Lane P, Kirmani JF, Ahmed S, Jacob M, Zada Y, Divani AA. Treatment of acute hypertension in patients with intracerebral hemorrhage using American Heart Association guidelines. Crit Care Med. 2006;34(7):1975–1980.

9. Anderson CS. Medical management of acute intracerebral hemorrhage. Curr Opin Crit Care. 2009;15(2):93–98.

10. Hemphill JC 3rd, Bonovich DC, Besmertis L, Manley GT, Johnston SC. The ICH score: a simple, reliable grading scale for intracerebral hemorrhage. Stroke. 2001;32(4):891–897.

11. Anderson CS, Heeley E, Huang Y, et al. Rapid blood-pressure lowering in patients with acute intracerebral hemorrhage. N Engl J Med. 2013;368(25):2355–2365.

12. Mayer SA, Brun NC, Begtrup K, et al. Efficacy and safety of recombinant activated factor VII for acute intracerebral hemorrhage. N Engl J Med. 2008;358(20):2127–2137.

13. Diringer MN, Skolnick BE, Mayer SA, et al. Risk of thromboembolic events in controlled trials of rFVIIa in spontaneous intracerebral hemorrhage. Stroke. 2008;39(3):850–856.

14. Mendelow AD, Gregson BA, Fernandes HM, et al. Early surgery versus initial conservative treatment in patients with spontaneous supratentorial intracerebral haematomas in the International Surgical Trial in Intracerebral Haemorrhage (STICH): a randomised trial. Lancet. 2005;365(9457):387–397.

15. Mendelow AD, Gregson BA, Rowan EN, Murray GD, Gholkar A, Mitchell PM. Early surgery versus initial conservative treatment in patients with spontaneous supratentorial lobar intracerebral haematomas (STICH II): a randomised trial. Lancet. 2013;382(9890):397–408.

Spinal cord injury

Mypinder S. Sekhon and
Donald E. Griesdale

Table 9.1 Spinal cord injury mechanisms

Mechanism	Description
Impact & compression	Trauma with cord compression from bone/disc/hematoma
Impact & transient compression	Impact with hyperextension
Distraction	Stretching or shearing of cord in axial plane
Transection	Secondary to penetrating trauma or severe distraction

Table 9.2 American Spinal Injury Association (ASIA)

Grade	Description	Deficit
A	Complete	No motor or sensory below lesion
B	Incomplete	No motor below lesion; sensory preserved
C	Incomplete	Motor preserved below lesion, > 50% muscle groups grade < 3 strength
D	Incomplete	Motor preserved below lesion, > 50% muscle groups grade > 3 strength
E	Normal	Normal

Motor grading 0 = flaccid, 1 = fasciculation, 2 = movement without gravity, 3 = movement against gravity only, 4 = decreased strength against active resistance, 5 = full strength against active resistance. Sensory grading (light tough, pin prick, temperature) 0 = absent, 1 = impaired, 2 = normal.

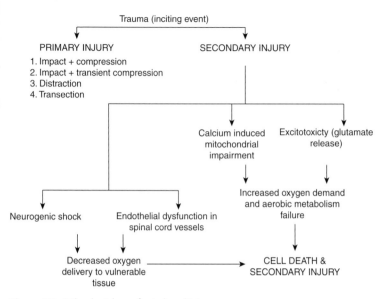

Figure 9.1 Pathophysiology of spinal cord injury.

Traumatic spinal cord injury

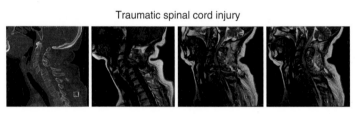

Figure 9.2 Traumatic spinal cord injury. Magnetic resonance imaging demonstrating retropulsion of a cervical vertebral body with impingement on the spinal cord.

Similar to TBI, the hemodynamic management of spinal cord injury focuses on the prevention of secondary ischemic injury. Once secondary ischemic injury ensues, a complex cascade of cellular dysfunction results in permanent damage of potentially viable tissue.

Table 9.3 Spinal cord syndromes

Syndrome	Etiology	Mechanism	Symptoms/signs
Acute central cord	Osteophyte compression & anterior Ligamentum flavum compression & posterior compression fractures and fracture dislocation	Hyperextension	Arms > legs weakness Pain/temp loss at level of lesion & intersects spinothalamic tract crossing
Anterior cord	Anterior dislocation/ compression fracture of vertebral body Malignancy Anterior spinal artery thrombosis/ dissection	Flexion/rotation	Bilateral pain/temp loss Symmetric motor weakness Potential arm sparring Intact light touch/ proprioception and vibration
Brown sequard	Penetrating injuries Lateral vertebral fractures	Hemisection of cord	Ipsilateral light touch/ proprioception/ vibtration loss Ipsilateral motor weakness Contralateral temp/pain loss
Cauda equina	Disc or bony protrusion of lumbar vertebra Malignancy	Compression of cauda equina by fracture or malignancy	Bowel/bladder incontinence Saddle anesthesia Leg numbness/weakness
Posterior cord	Fractures of posterior elements of vertebra	Hyperextension	Proprioception/ vibtration/light touch loss
Conus medullaris	Sacral fractures	Associated pelvic trauma	Sphincter dysfunction and sacral sensory loss

Table 9.4 Approach to causes of acute myeloptahy

Category	Subcategory	Specific etiology	Notes
Non-traumatic	Vascular	Anterior spinal cord syndrome	Dissection, embolic source is rare
		Posterior spinal cord syndrome	Occlusion of artery of Adamkowiecz
			Aortic dissection
		Dural AVM	
		Dural venous fistula	
	Autoimmune	See Table 9.5	
	Infectious	See Table 9.5	
	Malignancy	Bony metastasis from distant primary malignancy site.	Common metastatic malignancies: lung, breast, prostate, GI lymphoma
Traumatic	See Table 9.1.		

Transverse myelitis

Definition: Inflammatory damage of the spinal cord secondary to a primary etiology.

Table 9.5 Approach to the etiology of transverse myelitis

Category	Specific etiology	
Demyelinating	Multiple sclerosis, neuromyelitis optica, acute disseminated encephalomyelitis, post vaccine	
Inflammatory	SLE, Sjogren's, sarcoidosis, Behçet's, systemic sclerosis, mixed connective tissue disease	
Infectious	Viral	VZV, CMV, EBV, HSV, influenza A, measles, mumps, enteroviruses, flaviviruses, hepatitis A & C
	Bacterial	Treponema pallidum, Borrelia burgdorferi, mycobacterium tuberculosis
	Fungal	coccidiomycosis, blastomycosis, aspergillus, actinomyces,
	parasite	neurocysticercosis, schistosomiasis
Paraneoplastic	Anti-amphiphysin (breast), anti-CRMP 5 (small cell lung cancer)	

Table 9.6 Diagnostic criteria of transverse myelitis

Component	Criteria
Spinal cord involvement	Sensory/ motor autonomic dysfunction attributable to spinal cord
Distribution of symptoms	Bilateral signs or symptoms
Site of lesion	Clearly defined sensory level
Timing	Progression to nadir within 4 h to 21 days
Evidence of pathology	Evidence of spinal cord inflammation by gadolinium enhancement, CSF pleocytosis or elevated IgG index

Management

Table 9.7 Approach to traumatic spinal cord injury management

Approach		Intervention
Cord specific		Transfer to Level 1 trauma centre
		Immobilization
		a. C-spine, T-spine, L-spine
		b. Clearance of spines in consultation with spine service
		surgical decompression
		a. Within 24 h of admission
Complication management		
Respiratory	Pneumonia	Pneumonia detection & therapy
		a. Tracheal suction cultures + radiography
		b. Likely nosocomial infection & broad-spectrum antimicrobials
		Ventilator-associated pneumonia prevention bundle
		a. Chlorhexidine mouth wash
		b. EVAC endotracheal tube
		c. Head of bed 30°
		d. Tracheal suctioning
	Pulmonary Embolism	Deep vein thrombosis prevention
		a. Low molecular weight heparin (Enoxaparin)
		b. Early mobilization
	Pulmonary toilet	Bronchial hygeine management
		a. Tracheal suctioning
		b. Chest physiotherapy
		c. Therapeutic bronchoscopy
		d. Consider early tracheostomy

Table 9.7 (cont.)

Complication management

	Ventilation	Mechanical ventilation wean
		a. Determination of difficulty of wean
		– Complete vs. incomplete injury
		– Site of cord injury (upper C-spine vs. lower)
		b. Coordinated multidisciplinary weaning plan
		c. Consideration of abdominal binder to assist in weaning
Cardiovascular	Hemodynamic management	Neurogenic shock (esp. T1–T5 involvement)
		a. Vasopressors
		– Norepinephrine 1st line
		– Dopamine if chonotropy decreased
		Perfusion target
		a. Mean arterial pressure goal 80–85 mmHg for cord perfusion
Gastrointestinal		Nutrition
		a. Enteral route preferred, altered energy requirements
		Glucose control
		a. Insulin infusion protocol to aim for BG 6–10

Evidence-based neurocritical care

Table 9.8 The role of steroids in spinal cord injury

Question	The role of glucocorticoids in SCI
Summary	Two RCTs have examined the efficacy of methylprednisolone (MP) in patients with acute spinal cord injury. National Acute Spinal Cord Injury Study (NASCIS II) randomized 427 patients to MP, naloxone or placebo. Of uncertain clinical value, there was an improvement in motor scores in a subset of patients who received MP within 8 hours. NASCIS III RCT of 499 patients compared 24 h MP to 48 h MP and showed no improvement in neurologic function or mortality at 1 year. Longer duration of MP led to more sepsis and pneumonia. Based on these and other trials, updated guidelines from the American Association of Neurological Surgeons and the Congress of Neurological Surgeons did not recommend MP in acute spinal cord injury.

Summary

- Traumatic spinal cord injury occurs by four different mechanisms: transection, impact and compression, impact and transient compression and distraction.
- Diagnosis of SCI requires prompt physical examination and magnetic resonance imaging.
- Management of SCI focuses on decompression of the SCI, monitoring for complications and treating them in the intensive care unit.

Suggested readings

1. Jia X, Kowalski R, Sciubba D, Geocadin RG. Critical care of traumatic spinal cord injury. J Intensive Care Med. 2013;28:12.

2. Maynard F, Bracken M, Creasey G, et al. International standards for neurological and functional classification of spinal cord injury. Spinal Cord. 1995;35:266–274.

3. Furlan JC, Noonan V, Cadotte DW, Fehlings M. Timing of decompressive surgery of spinal cord after traumatic spinal cord injury: An evidence based examination of preclinical and clinical studies. J Neurotrauma. 2011;28:1371–1399.

4. Dimar JR, Carreon L, Riina J, et al. Early vs. late stabilization of the spine in the polytrauma patient. Spine. 2010; 35:187–192.

5. Bracken MB, Shepard MJ, Collins WF, et al. Methylprednisolone or naloxone treatment after acute spinal cord injury: 1-year follow-up data. Results of the second National Acute Spinal Cord Injury Study. J Neurosurg. 1992;76(1):23–31.

6. Bracken MB, Shepard MJ, Holford TR, et al. Methylprednisolone or tirilazad mesylate administration after acute spinal cord injury: 1-year follow up. Results of the third National Acute Spinal Cord Injury randomized controlled trial. J Neurosurg. 1998;89(5):699–706.

7. Hurlbert RJ, Hadley MN, Walters BC, et al. Pharmacological therapy for acute spinal cord injury. Neurosurgery. 2013;72(Suppl 2):93–105.

Chapter 10

Hydrocephalus

Mypinder S. Sekhon and
Donald E. Griesdale

Definition: A disturbance of cerebral spinal fluid formation, flow or absorption resulting in enlarged cerebral spinal fluid compartment within the central nervous system.

A. Communicating hydrocephalus: Hydrocephalus with full communication between the ventricular system and the subarachnoid space. It is usually caused by ineffective CSF absorption or excess CSF production.

B. Non-communicating hydrocephalus: Hydrocephalus results from an obstruction of CSF flow within the path of the ventricular system or its outlets.

C. Normal pressure hydrocephalus: Hydrocephalus occurring in predominantly elderly patients who exhibit normal intracranial pressure, in spite of increased CSF compartment size.

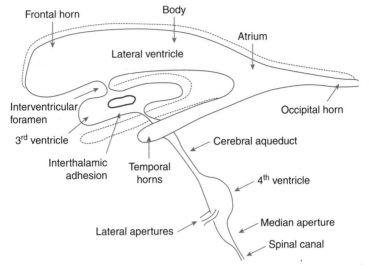

Figure 10.1 Anatomy of the cerebral ventricular system. Both lateral ventricles drain cerebral spinal fluid (CSF) into the 3rd ventricle via the interventricular foramen (foramen of Monro). The 3rd ventricle drains into the 4th ventricle via the cerebral aqueduct (aqueduct of Sylvius). CSF exits the 4th ventricle via the lateral and median apertures (Lushka and Magendie, respectively). Thereafter, it enters the spinal canal or circulates to the superior sagittal sinus where it is absorbed into the sagittal venous sinus through arachnoid granulations.

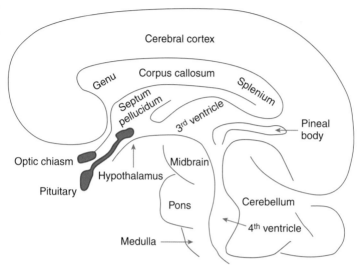

Figure 10.2 Sagittal anatomy of the cerebrum and brainstem. The anatomy of the ventricular system is demonstrated alongside major anatomical structures of the central nervous system. Importantly, the 4th ventricle lies between the cerebellum and brainstem, a narrow area where obstruction to CSF flow can occur, resulting in non-communicating hydrocephalus.

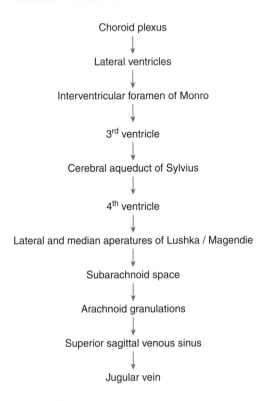

Choroid plexus

↓

Lateral ventricles

↓

Interventricular foramen of Monro

↓

3rd ventricle

↓

Cerebral aqueduct of Sylvius

↓

4th ventricle

↓

Lateral and median aperatures of Lushka / Magendie

↓

Subarachnoid space

↓

Arachnoid granulations

↓

Superior sagittal venous sinus

↓

Jugular vein

Figure 10.3 Cerebral spinal fluid path of flow. CSF production occurs at approximately 0.2–0.35 ml/min in the choroid plexi of the lateral and 4th ventricles. Approximately 30 ml of CSF is contained within the lateral and 3rd ventricles. There is a total of ~ 120ml of CSF at any one point. CSF production usually decreases in states of increased ICP.

Table 10.1 Diagnostic considerations for hydrocephalus

Imaging modality	Utility
CT	Assess ventricular size and determine communicating vs. non-communicating
MRI	Assess for underlying lesion causing hydrocephalus–superior visualization for: A. Cerebellar tumors B. Posterior fossa C. Chiari malformation D. Periaqueductal tumor
Imaging criteria	1. Temporal horn size > 2 mm. Normally temporal horns should only be barely visible. 2. Largest frontal horn diameter: largest biparietal diameter ratio > 30%. 3. Periventricular hypoattentuation (CT) or hyperintensity on T2 (MRI): transependymal exudate. 4. Upward bowing of corpus callosum on sagittal MRI suggests acute hydrocephalus. 5. Frontal horn and 3rd ventricle enlargement suggests cerebral aqueduct obstruction.

Computed tomography demonstrating non-communicating hydrocephalus

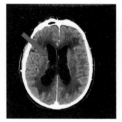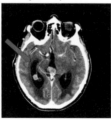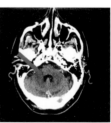

Figure 10.4 **CT evidence of non-communicating hydrocephalus.** Adjacent to the dilated lateral ventricles, periventricular edema is shown stemming from increased intraventricular pressures.

Table 10.2 Surgical and medical management of hydrocephalus

Approach	Intervention	Notes
Surgical	**Shunts**	
	Ventroperitoneal	Most common. Diverts CSF from lateral ventricles to peritoneal cavity.
	Ventroarterial	Diverts CSF from lateral ventricles to right atrium through jugular vein and superior vena cava. Reserved for patients with abdominal pathology (malignancy, peritonitis, major abdominal surgery).
	Lumboperitoneal	Only can be used in communicating hydrocephalus.
	Ventropleural	Second line. Used if other shunts are contraindicated.
	Torkildsen shunt	Diverts CSF from lateral ventricles to cisternal space. Rarely used.
	External ventricular drain	Used in acute hydrocephalus as emergent procedure.
	Other	
	Endoscopic 3rd ventriculostomy	Alternative route for CSF diversion. Can be completed by endoscopic puncture of the 3rd ventricle floor.
	Cerebral aqueductoplasty	Useful if tumor resection occurring simultaneously.
	Choroid plexectomy	Reserved for refractory cases. Laser coagulation of choroid plexus.
	Lumbar puncture	Can only be done in communicating hydrocephalus.
Medical	Acetazolamide Furosemide	Controversial. Both diuretics appear to decrease the production of CSF at the level of the choroid plexus.

Summary

- Hydrocephalus is a state of abnormal CSF production, flow or absorption, resulting in an enlarged CSF compartment.
- Communicating hydrocephalus most commonly occurs from decreased CSF absorption or increased production. The flow of CSF is intact.
- Non-communicating hydrocephalus occurs from an obstruction to CSF flow within the ventricular system or its outlets.
- Diagnosis requires careful history/examination and imaging, demonstrating an enlarged ventricular system.
- Management of hydrocephalus is predominantly surgical with shunt therapy as its mainstay.

Suggested readings

1. Fishman MA. Hydrocephalus. In Neurological Pathophysiology, Eliasson SG, Prensky AL, Hardin WB (Eds.), New York: Oxford, 1978.

2. Carey CM, Tullous MW, Walker ML. Hydrocephalus: Etiology, pathologic effects, diagnosis, and natural history. In Pediatric Neurosurgery, 3rd edn, Cheek WR (Ed.), Philadelphia: WB Saunders Company, 1994.

3. Akins PT, Guppy KH, Axelrod YV, et al. The genesis of low pressure hydrocephalus. Neurocrit Care 2011; 15:461.

4. Rekate HL. Treatment of hydrocephalus. In Pediatric Neurosurgery, 3rd edn, Cheek WR (Ed.), Philadelphia: WB Saunders Company, 1994.

5. Kirkpatrick M, Engleman H, Minns RA. Symptoms and signs of progressive hydrocephalus. Arch Dis Child 1989; 64:124.

Chapter

11

Ischemic stroke

Mypinder S. Sekhon and Manraj Heran

Ischemic injury to cerebral tissue secondary to insufficient cerebral oxygen delivery from vascular occlusion or compromise.

Etiology

Table 11.1 Approach to etiology of ischemic stroke

Category	Frequency	Mechanism	Etiology
Embolic	70%	Vessel to vessel	Aortic arch or carotid plaque rupture
		Cardioembolic	Atrial fibrillation with left atrial clot
			Valvular vegetation
			Left ventricular aneurysm with apical clot
			Atrial myxoma
			Paradoxical (right to left clot transit via shunt)
Thrombotic	25%	Lacunar	Intracranial arteriolar thrombosis
			Associated with DM/HTN/ cerebrovascular disease
Other	5%	Arterial dissection	Most common sites: carotid or vertebral
			Secondary to trauma most commonly
		Vasospasm	Post aneurysmal SAH
			Post traumatic brain injury
			Vasospastic diseases
		Vasculitis	Systemic lupus erythematosis
			Sarcoidosis

Table 11.1 (cont.)

Category	Frequency	Mechanism	Etiology
		Hyperviscosity	Erythrocytes: polycythemia rubra vera
			Leukocytes: myeloid hematologic malignancy
			Serum proteins: Waldenstrom's macroglobulinemia, MM
		Watershed	Any cause of prolonged global hypotension

Diagnosis

Table 11.2 Imaging modalities and utility in ischemic stroke

Imaging modality	Rationale
Non-contrast CT	Rule out hemorrhagic stroke
CT angiogram	Delineate vascular anatomy/patency
MRI	High sensitivity for cerebral infarction
CT perfusion	Establish areas of reversible ischemia

Early MCA ischemia   MCA occlusion   Malignant edema

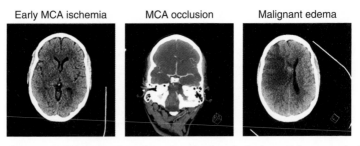

Figure 11.1 MCA ischemic stroke and resultant cerebral edema. Malignant cerebral edema can result after a large MCA stroke, which can cause intracranial herniation syndromes.

Basilar artery occlusion

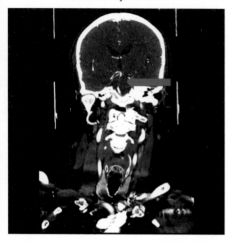

Figure 11.2 Computed tomography angiogram of basilar artery thrombosis. CT angiogram revealing acute basilar artery thrombosis.

Table 11.3 Clinical signs and symptoms of stroke syndromes

Artery	Clinical signs/symptoms
ICA	Monocular blindness Contralateral extremity hemiplegia/hemianesthesia (leg = arm = face) Dominant hemisphere – aphasia Non-dominant hemisphere – apraxia & neglect
Opthalmic	Monocular visual impairment
MCA	Contralateral extremity hemiplegia/hemianesthesia (arm/face > leg) Dominant hemisphere – expressive aphasia Non-dominant hemisphere – apraxia & neglect Homonymous hemianopsia
ACA	Contralateral extremity hemiplegia/hemianesthesia (leg > arm/face) Primitive reflexes Urinary incontinence
PCA	Macular-sparing homonymous hemianopsia Thalamic syndromes Contralateral hemianesthesia Dominant hemisphere – receptive aphasia
Basilar	Symmetric quadriplegia/sensory loss

Table 11.3 (cont.)

Artery	Clinical signs/symptoms
	Cranial nerve abnormalities Altered level of consciousness
Vertebral	Wallenburg's syndrome – ipsilateral face & contraleteral extremity Hemianesthesia Diplopia Dysarthria Ipsilateral Horner's syndrome

(Adapted from *Pocket Medicine*, 3rd edition, 2008, Lippincott Williams and Wilkins.)

Right MCA   Basilar   CTA of basilar   PCA

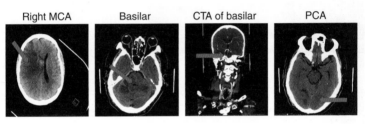

Figure 11.3 CT imaging of stroke syndromes.

Etiologic diagnostics

Table 11.4 Investigations in evaluation of ischemic stroke

Diagnostic test	Specific tests	Notes
General labs	CBC Renal profile INR/PTT	Baseline, thrombocytopenia as CI for thrombolysis Baseline Coagulopathy CI for thrombolysis
Echocardiogram	Transthoracic Transesophageal Bubble Study	Evaluate for LV aneurysm, vegetations, myxoma *Consider* TEE for left-atrium appendage clot with atrial fibrillation Right to left shunt evaluation

Table 11.4 (cont.)

Diagnostic test	Specific tests	Notes
Electrocardiographic	Holter	Evaluation for paroxysmal A. Fib.
Ultrasonography	Carotid Doppler	Etiologic diagnosis of carotid artery embolism

CBC = Complete blood count, INR = International normalized ratio, PTT = Prothrombin time,
CI = Contraindication, LV = Left ventricle, TEE = transesophageal echocardiography.

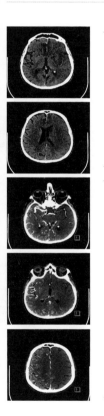

Non-contrast CT showing early MCA ischemia

CT angiogram demonstrating absent MCA blood flow

Figure 11.4 Non-contrast and CT angiogram demonstrating the appearance of early ischemia with corresponding absent blood flow on angiography.

Management

Table 11.5 Approach to management of ischemic stroke

Approach	Treatment	Notes	Evidence
Revascularization	Thrombolysis	Indications a. Within 4.5 h of symptom onset b. Large deficit c. Basilar artery thrombosis within 24 h Contraindications a. Concomitant ICH b. Previous ICH c. BP > 180/110 mmHg d. Head trauma/stroke < 3 months e. Intracranial lesion (neoplasm, aneurysm, AVM) f. Active bleeding or coagulopathy g. Trauma/surgery within < 3 weeks h. > 33% of hemisphere ischemic Dose a. 0.9 mg/kg IV with 10% bolus over 1 min then remaining over 1 hour	12 % ↑ functional outcome 4% ↓ ARR death 5% ↑ risk of ICH
	Intra-arterial therapy	Indication a. Large-vessel occlusion – proximal clot. Mechanical clot extraction has possible additional benefit	Negative RCTs for IA lysis Clot extraction not yet evaluated in RCTs
Medical therapy	Hemodynamic	Post thrombolysis: < 180/105 mmHg No thrombolysis: < 220/120 mmHg Agents a. Beta blockers b. Ca channel blockers c. ACEI/ARB d. Vasodilators – Hydralazine	Grade 2A Grade 2A Grade 1C Grade 2B Grade 1A Grade 2B

Table 11.5 (cont.)

Approach	Treatment	Notes	Evidence
	DVT Proph.	Enoxaparin > SC heparin in DVT prevention in ischemic stroke pts	Grade 1A
	2° prevention	Antiplatelet a. ASA + dyprimadole > ASA alone	↓ death/stroke Grade 1A ↑ repeat stroke
		Lipid-lowering a. High-dose statin	
Complications	Cerebral edema	Refer to increased ICP protocol Decompressive craniectomy	NNT 3 for death in malignant edema
	Seizure	Refer for status epilepticus protocol Establish continuous EEG	10% incidence of seizures
	Hemorrhagic transformation	Refer to ICH protocol	1–2% risk overall, higher post-tPA

ICH = intracerebral hemorrhage, AVM = arteriovenous malformation, ARR = absolute risk reduction, RCT = randomized control lead trial, ACEI = angiotensin converting enzyme inhibitor, ARB = angiotensin receptor blocker, DVT = deep vein thrombosis, SC = subcutaneous, ASA = acetylsalicyclic acid, NNT = number needed to treat, ICP = intracranial pressure, EEG = electroencephalogram, tPA = tissue plasminogen activator.

Evidence-based neurocritical care

Table 11.6 The IST trial

Title	The International Stroke Trial (IST): a randomized trial of aspirin, subcutaneous heparin, both, or neither among 19,435 patients with acute ischaemic stroke. International Stroke Trial Collaborative Group.
Summary	IST was a large, multicenter 2×3 factorial RCT of 19,435 patients comparing ASA 300 mg to no ASA in the following three groups: heparin 12,500 U b.i.d, heparin 5,000 U b.i.d and placebo. Patients allocated to ASA had fewer recurrent ischemic strokes within 14 days (2.8% vs. 3.9%) without an increase in hemorrhagic strokes. Patients allocated to heparin also had fewer recurrent ischemic strokes (2.9% vs. 3.8%) but this benefit was negated by an increase in hemorrhagic strokes (1.2% vs. 0.4%).

Table 11.7 The role of tPA in acute ischemic stroke

Title	Tissue plasminogen activator for acute ischemic stroke. The National Institute of Neurological Disorders and Stroke rt-PA Stroke Study Group
Summary	NINDS was an RCT of 624 patients. Overall, t-PA given within 180 minutes improved favourable outcome at 3 months (34% vs. 21%); t-PA also increased the risk of fatal and non-fatal ICH (7% vs. 1%). The window of 3 hours has been subsequently extended to 4.5 h based on the ECASS III trial, which confirmed the favourable outcome in 821 patients who received t-PA between 3 and 4.5 h (52% vs. 45%, p = 0.04).

Table 11.8 The role of intra-arterial therapy in ischemic stroke.

Title	Efficacy of intra-arterial fibrinolysis for acute ischemic stroke: meta-analysis of randomized controlled trials.
Summary	Meta-analysis of 5 RCTs with 395 patients compared intra-arterial thrombolysis + IV heparin to IV heparin alone. Overall, IA thrombolysis was associated with increased good outcome (42% vs. 28%) but increased risk of symptomatic ICH (31% vs. 18%). The majoirty of the patients included in the meta-analyses were contributed from the PROACT II study, which randomized 180 patients with MCA occlusion. IA thrombolysis increased the likelihood of a good outcome (40% vs. 25%). Thus, patients who have large-vessel occlusion (e.g., MCA or basilar artery) or who have a contra-indication to IV-tPA may be reasonable candidates for IA thrombolysis.

Summary

- Ischemic stroke results from inadequate oxygen supply to a specific vascular region of the cerebral parenchyma. Common etiologies include vessel to vessel emboli or cardiogenic emboli.
- Prompt diagnosis requires a focussed neurological physical exam, computed tomography and cerebral angiography.
- If diagnosed quickly, it is imperative to establish reperfusion of the culprit occluded artery with thrombolysis and thereafter preventing repeat stroke by risk stratification and medical therapy.

Suggested readings

1. De Georgia M, Patel V. Critical care management in acute ischemic stroke. J Neurointerv Surg. 2011 Mar;3(1):34–7.

2. Bernstein RA, Hemphill JC. Critical care of acute ischemic stroke. Curr Neurol Neurosci Rep. 2001 Nov;1(6):587–92.

3. Finley Caulfield A, Wijman CA. Critical care of acute ischemic stroke. Crit Care Clin. 2006 Oct;22(4):581–606.

4. Finley Caulfield A, Wijman CA. Management of acute ischemic stroke. Neurol Clin. 2008 May;26(2):345–71.

5. Lewandowski C, Barsan W. Treatment of acute ischemic stroke. Ann Emerg Med. 2001 Feb;37(2):202–16

6. The International Stroke Trial (IST): a randomised trial of aspirin, subcutaneous heparin, both, or neither among 19,435 patients with acute ischaemic stroke. International Stroke Trial Collaborative Group. Lancet. 1997;349(9065):1569–81.

7. Tissue plasminogen activator for acute ischemic stroke. The National Institute of Neurological Disorders and Stroke rt-PA Stroke Study Group. N Engl J Med. 1995;333(24):1581–7.

8. Hacke W, Kaste M, Bluhmki E, et al. Thrombolysis with alteplase 3 to 4.5 hours after acute ischemic stroke. N Engl J Med. 2008;359(13):1317–29.

9. Lee M, Hong K-S, Saver JL. Efficacy of intra-arterial fibrinolysis for acute ischemic stroke: meta-analysis of randomized controlled trials. Stroke. 2010;41(5):932–7.

10. Furlan A, Higashida R, Wechsler L, et al. Intra-arterial prourokinase for acute ischemic stroke. The PROACT II study: a randomized controlled trial. Prolyse in Acute Cerebral Thromboembolism. JAMA. 1999;282(21):2003–11.

Status epilepticus

Mypinder S. Sekhon

Status epilepticus: Clinical or electrographic seizures of > 5 minutes or recurrent seizure activity without recovery in between episodes.

Refractory status epileptcus: Persistent clinical or electrographic seizures despite benzodiazepines and one anti epileptic drug (AED).

Etiology

Table 12.1 Approach to etiology of status epilepticus

Category	Specific etiologies
Drugs	Non-compliance with AEDs Overdose – Salicylates, sympathomimetics, isoniazid Withdrawal of alcohol, benzodiazepines, other sedatives Psychotropic medications – especially anticholinergics
Infection	Meningitis/encephalitis – especially HSV Intracranial abscess
Metabolic	Electrolyte disturbance – Na^+, Mg^{2+}, Ca^{2+} Renal failure/uremia, fulminant liver failure Hypoglycemia
Structural	Neoplasm, traumatic brain injury, degenerative neurologic disease
Stroke/Vascular	Ischemic stroke, intracerebral hemorrhage, subarachnoid hemorrhage cerebral sinus thrombosis
Other	Autoimmune antibodies, paraneoplastic antibodies Post cardiac arrest, hypertensive emergency

Pathophysiology

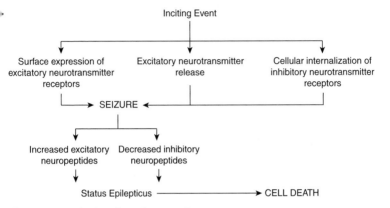

Figure 12.1 Pathophysiology of status epilepticus.

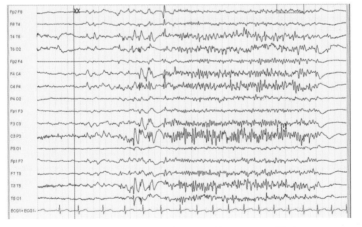

Figure 12.2 Electroencephalograhy of status epilepticus post TBI. Active seizures are shown on continuous EEG readings in patients post TBI. The incidence of seziures in this population can vary from 20–40%.

Table 12.2 Suggested diagnostic work-up

Status epilepticus

Investigations	CBC, electrolytes (incl. Mg^{2+}, Ca^{2+}, PO_4^{3-}) & glucose Urea/Cr + liver enzymes and function AED serum levels, if applicable Toxicology screen – serum + urine
Imaging	CT head with and without contrast +/– MRI

Additional investigations	Continuous EEG
	Lumbar puncture – CSF investigations:
	1. Gram stain, culture, virology (esp. HSV PCR)
	2. Chemistry
	3. Cell count + differential
	4. Save for additional investigations
	   a. VDRL, cryptococcal Ag, TB PCR, AFB
	   b. Oligoclonal banding (MS, Lyme disease,
	      autoimmune disease, solid and
	      lymphoproliferative malignancy, GBS).

Refractory status epilepticus

Imaging	MRI head with GAD. *Consider* repeat MRI in 5–7days if etiology unknown or for disease evolution
Antibody-mediated encephalitis (autoimmune vs. paraneoplastic)	Obtain serum levels: 1. Anti-NMDA, anti-Yo/Ri 2. Anti-VGKC, anti-LGI1 3. Anti-Hu, anti-Ma2, anti-NMO 4. Anti-CRMP5, anti-CASPR2 5. Anti-AMPAR, anti-$GABA^B$ Malignancy evaluation: 1. CT chest, abdomen, pelvis 2. Pelvic US or testicular US 3. Bronchoscopy, endoscopy, colonoscopy 4. Serum tumor markers
Vasculitis/autoimmune	ANA, ENA panel, complement levels

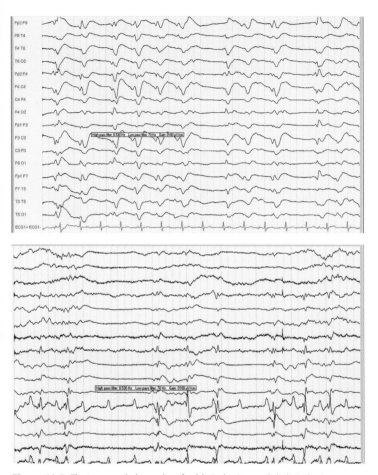

Figure 12.3 **Electroencephalography of sublinical seizures**. Subclinical seizures are defined by the lack of physical manifestations of seizure-like activity. In the critically ill population, the vast majority of seizures in patients are non-convulsive or sublinical, making EEG monitoring necessary for diagnosis and evaluation.

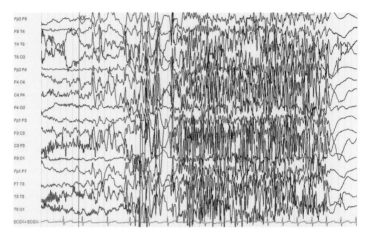

Figure 12.4 EEG revealing non-convulsive status epilepticus. The seizures are not focally located and generalized seizure activity is seen throughout all channels.

Limbic encephalitis - HSV

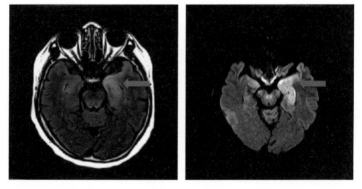

Figure 12.5 Magnetic resonance imaging of limbic encephalitis. Paraneoplastic and autoimmune-mediated antibody production can lead to selective involvement of the temporal lobes resulting in limbic encephalitis.

Table 12.3 Antibody-mediated status epilepticus

Category	Antibody	Associations	MRI findings
Autoimmune	Anti-VGKC	Autoimmune	LE
	Anti-NMO	Neuromyelitis optica	RE, optic nerve

Category	Antibody	Site of Malignancy	MRI findings
Paraneoplastic	Anti-NMDA	Ovarian	LE or normal
	Anti-Hu	Lung, neuroblastoma	LE, RE, DE
	Anti-Ma2	Testicular, lung, breast	LE, RE, DE
	Anti-CASPR2	Thymus, uterine	LE
	Anti-CRMP5	Lung, thymoma	LE, CE, SE
	Anti-LGI1	Lung, thyroid, renal, thymus	LE, normal
	Anti-GABA^B	Lung	LE, normal
	Anti-AMPAR	Lung, breast	LE
	Anti-Yo	Ovarian, breast, uterine	CE
	Anti-Ri	Ovarian, breast, neuroblastoma, lung	RE, CE

LE = Limbic encephalitis, RE = Rhomboencephalitis, DE = Diencephalon encephalitis, CE = Cerebellar encephalitis, SE = Striatal encephalitis.

Management

Status epilepticus: Clinical or electrographic seizures of > 5 mins or recurrent seizure activity without recovery in between episodes
Refractory status epileptcus: Persistent clinical or electrographic seizures despite benzodiazepines and one anti epileptic drug

Airway protection & anti epileptic therapy
Evaluate for underlying cause

LEVEL 1: Status epilepticus

1. Lorazepam 0.1 mg/kg IV, repeat × 3 if necessary, or midazolam 0.2 mg/kg IV, repeat × 3 if necessary
2. Phenytoin 20 mg/kg IV load, then 5–7 mg/kg IV every 8 hours

If clinical or electrographic seizures continue despite Level 1 therapy for > 5 mins then proceed to Level 2

LEVEL 2 - Refractory status epilepticus

1. Propofol 1–2 mg/kg IV bolus, then 0–80 mcg/kg/min IV infusion and/or
2. Midazolam 0.2 mg/kg IV bolus, then 0.05–2 mg/kg/h IV infusion and/or
3. Valproic acid 20–30 mg/kg IV load, then 10 mg/kg/d divided in 2–3 doses daily

Consider additional anti epileptic therapy:
1. Levetiracetam 500–1500 mg twice daily
2. Topiramate 200–400 mg/d, titrate to 400–1600 mg daily
3. Pregabalin 50 mg three times daily
4. Clonazepam 0.5–2 mg twice daily
5. Lacosamide 200–400 IV daily

Establish continuous EEG monitoring
If clinical or electrographic seizures persist then proceed to Level 3

LEVEL 3 - Alternative therapies

1. Ketamine 1.5–3 mg/kg IV bolus, then 1–5 mg/kg/h IV infusion and/or
2. Pentobarbital 10 mg/kg IV load then 0.5–2 mg/kg/h IV infusion

Maintain continuous EEG monitoring
Maintain IV anti epileptic therapy for 24–48 h with EEG complete seizure cessation
or burst suppression
Wean off intravenous therapies

Other treatments:
Therapeutic hypothermia (temp 35–36°C)
Consider surgical resection – if single electrographic focus established
Magnesium – 20 mmol IV load over 4 h then 10–30 mmol/h infusion. Target serum
Mg^{2+} 3.5 mmol/L
Ketogenic diet
Electroconvulsive therapy

Table 12.4 Antiepileptic medications and associated adverse effects

Antiepileptic medication	Organ system	Side effects/adverse reactions
Phenytoin	Hepatic	Transaminitis
	Derm	Steven Johnson's, gingival hypertrophy
	Heme	Megaloblastic anemia
	Endo	Adrenal insufficiency
Levetiracetam	Hepatic	Mild transaminitis

Table 12.4 (cont.)

Antiepileptic medication	Organ system	Side effects/adverse reactions
Valproic acid	Hepatic	Transaminitis, fulminant hepatic failure, hyperammonemia
	Heme	Thrombocyopenia
	Derm	Alopecia
Phenobarbital	Cardiac	Hypotension with intravenous administration
	Derm	Rash
	Heme	Macrocytic anemia, folate deficiency
Carbamazepine	Heme	Thrombocytopenia, leukopenia, aplastic anemia
	Renal	Hyponatremia – SIADH
Topiramate	Derm	Rash
Clonazepam	CNS	Altered level of consciousness, sedation
Lacosamide	CNS	Sedation, tremor

Summary

- Status epilepticus is a disease which, if not treated aggressively, can lead to continued seizures and neuronal damage.
- The diagnosis of SE involves the use of EEG and in-depth investigation evaluating the cause of SE.
- There are numerous emerging antibody-mediated causes of SE, which can be autoimmune in etiology or paraneoplastic.
- The management of SE involves treating the underlying condition and the use of multiple antiepileptic agents to terminate seizures under the guidance of continuous EEG.

Suggested readings

1. Brophy GM, Bell R, Classen J, Alldrege B et al. Guidelines for the evaluation and management of status epilepticus. Neurocrit Care. 2012;17(1):3–23.

2. Rosetti A, Lowenstein RH. Management of refractory status epilepticus in adults: still more questions than answers. Lancet Neurol. 2011;10:922–930.

3. Fernandez A, Claasen J. Refractory status epilepticus. Curr Opin Crit Care. 2011;18(2):127–135.

4. Chen JWY, Wasterlain C. Status epilepticus: pathophysiology and management in adults. Lancet Neurol. 2006;5:246–256.

5. Kowalski RG, Ziai WC, Rees RN, Werner JK, et al. Third-line antiepileptic therapy and outcome in status epilepticus: The impact of vasopressor use and prolonged mechanical ventilation. Crit Care Med. 2012;40:2677–2688.

Chapter 13

Neuromuscular disorders

Mypinder S. Sekhon

Dysfunction in one or multiple components of the nerve–muscle pathway resulting in weakness.

Etiology

Table 13.1 Anatomical approach to neuromuscular weakness and etiologies

Site	Etiology	
Brain	Vascular	Ischemic or hemorrhagic CVA
	Malignancy	Primary or metastasis
	Infection	Encephalitis
	Autoimmune/inflammatory	Multiple sclerosis
		Vasculidities
Spinal cord	Focal lesion	Trauma, hemorrhage, ischemia
		Malignancy
		Infection
	Diffuse	Transverse myelitis
		– Viral (CMV, VZV, HIV)
		– Multiple sclerosis
		– Autoimmune
		– Idiopathic
Anterior Horn	Acute	Poliomyelitis
	Chronic	Post polio
		ALS
Peripheral nerve	Demyelinating	Acute – GBS
		Subacute – see Table 13.2
		Chronic – see Table 13.2
	Axonal	Acute – vasculitis, porphyria
		Subacute – see Table 13.2
		Chronic – see Table 13.2
Neuromuscular junction	Antibody-induced	Myasthenia gravis
		Lambert–Eaton
	Infectious	Botulism
Muscle	Hereditary	Duchenne
		Becker
		Limb girdle
		Myotonic
	Inflammatory	Dermatomyositis, polymyositis, inclusion body myositis
	Endocrine	Cushing's hypothyroid
	Toxin/meds	Corticosteroids, statins, fibrates, colchicine, cocaine, anti-malarials

Table 13.2 Approach to peripheral neuropathy

Demyelinating		Axonal	
Acute	Guillain–Barré syndrome	Acute	Porphyria, vasculitis
Subacute	Taxol CIDP	Subacute	Meds: cisplatin, vincristine, INH Alcohol B12 deficiency

Chronic	Endo: DM, Hypothyroid
	Neoplasm: Paraneoplastic,
	  Myeloma, Waldenstrom's
	Critical illness polyneuropathy
		Chronic	DM
			Uremia
			Toxins: lead, arsenic
			Infection: Lyme, HIV
			Neoplasm: paraneoplastic,
			  myeloma, Waldenstrom's

CIDP = Chronic inflammatory demyelinating polyneuropathy, DM = Diabetes mellitus, INH = Isoniazid, HIV = Human immunodeficiency virus.
(Adapted from *Pocket Medicine*, 3rd edition, 2008, Lippincott Williams and Wilkins.)

Table 13.3 Approach to disorders of the neuromuscular junction

Myasthenia gravis vs. Lambert–Eaton		
Features	**Myasthenia gravis**	**Lambert–Eaton**
Clinical	Fatiguability	Paradoxical increased strength with repetition
Pathophysiology	Ab to post synaptic Ach receptor	Ab to presynaptic Ca^{2+} channel receptor
Associations	Thymoma	Small cell lung cancer

Diagnosis	Clinical: fatiguability
	Antibodies: anti-AchR,
	  anti-Musk
	EMG: decreased strength with
	  stimulation
		Clinical: increased strength with
		  repetition
		Antibodies: anti-VGCC
		EMG: increased strength with
		  stimulation

Treatment	See Table 13.5	Treat underlying disorder Immunomodulation

EMG = Electromyography, Ab = Antibody.

Table 13.4 Clinical distinguishing features of neuromuscular disease etiology

Clinical feature	Upper motor neuron	Lower motor neuron	Neuromuscular junction	Myopathy
Distribution	Regional	Distal	Proximal, symmetric	Proximal, symmetric
Atrophy	None	Severe	None	Mild
Fasiculation	None	Common	None	None
Tone	Increased	Decreased	Normal	Normal
Reflexes	Hyper-reflexia	Decreased/absent	Normal	Normal
Plantar reflex	Present	Absent	Absent	Absent
Sensation	Impaired if lesion located in: – sensory cortex – spinothalamic tract – dorsal columns	Stocking–glove distribution in demyelinating peripheral neuropathy (GBS etc.)	Normal	Normal

(Adapted from *Pocket Medicine*, 3rd edition, 2008, Lippincott Williams and Wilkins.)

Diagnosis

Table 13.5 Specific management principles of myasthenia gravis and Guillain–Barré syndrome

Disease	Treatment
Guillain–Barré syndrome	Treat precipitant Antibody sequestration/removal a. Plasmapheresis b. IVIG Mechanical ventilation a. Indications: VC < 20 ml/kg, MIP < 30 cm H_2O, MEP < 40 cm H_2O, progressive or decompensated hypercapnic respiratory failure, severe dysphagia with high risk of unprotected airway/aspiration b. Complete daily assessment for intubation and avoid extremis scenario Autonomic instability – cardiac monitoring and supportive care

Table 13.5 (cont.)

Disease	Treatment
Myasthenia gravis	Treat precipitant a. Removal of thymoma or thymus (effective in 85% of cases) Avoid medications that will precipitate myasthenic crisis Differentiate cholinergic excess from myasthenic crisis if on pyridostigmine Consider acetylcholinesterase inhibitor – pyridostigmine Immunomodulation a. High-dose corticosteroids – monitor for interval worsening b. Azathioprine or cyclophosphamide Antibody sequestration/removal a. Plasmapheresis b. IVIG Mechanical ventilation a. Indications: VC < 20 ml/kg, MIP < 30 cm H_2O, MEP < 40 cm H_2O, progressive or decompensated hypercapnic respiratory failure b. Complete daily assessment for intubation and avoid extremis scenario

IVIG = Intravenous immunoglobulin, VC = Vital capacity.

Management

Table 13.6 The role of plasmapheresis vs. IVIG in GBS

Question	Definitive therapy in GBS
Summary	In patients with Guillain–Barré syndrome, intravenous immuno globulin (IVIG) appears as effective as plama exchange. However, there appears to be no benefit in combining IVIG and plasmapharesis.

Summary

- Etiologies of neuromuscular dysfunction in the ICU patient can occur anywhere from the site of the central nervous system neuron, through the peripheral nerves, neuromuscular junction and to the muscle end plate.
- The clinical examination and EMG provide the key to differentiating the underlying causes of neuromuscular disease.
- The management strategy is unique for each etiology of neuromuscular dysfunction, making the diagnosis of the underlying condition imperative.
- Myasthenia gravis and Guillain–Barré syndrome are two distinct etiologies of neuromomuscular disease which have unique management strategies and are commonly seen in the intensive care setting.

Suggested readings

1. Sakaguchi H, Yamashita S, Hirano T. Myasthenic crisis patients who require intensive care unit management. Muscle Nerve. 2012 Sep;46(3):440–2.

2. Lacomis D. Myasthenic crisis. Neurocrit Care. 2005;3(3):189–94.

3. Juel VC. Myasthenia gravis: management of myasthenic crisis and perioperative care. Semin Neurol. 2004 Mar;24(1):75–81.

4. Hughes RA, Pritchard J, Hadden RD. Pharmacological treatment other than corticosteroids, intravenous immunoglobulin and plasma exchange for Guillain-Barré syndrome. Cochrane Database Syst Rev. 2013 Feb 28;2:CD008630.

5. McDaneld LM, Fields JD, Bourdette DN, Bhardwaj A. Immunomodulatory therapies in neurologic critical care. NeurocritCare. 2010 Feb;12(1):132–43.

6. Green DM. Weakness in the ICU: Guillain-Barré syndrome, myasthenia gravis, and critical illness polyneuropathy/myopathy. Neurologist. 2005 Nov;11(6):338–47.

7. Marinelli WA, Leatherman JW. Neuromuscular disorders in the intensive care unit. Crit Care Clin. 2002 Oct;18(4):915–29.

8. Dhand UK. Clinical approach to the weak patient in the intensive care unit. Respir Care. 2006 Sep;51(9):1024–40; discussion 1040–1.

9. Van der Meché FG, Schmitz PI. A randomized trial comparing intravenous immune globulin and plasma exchange in Guillain-Barré syndrome. Dutch Guillain-Barré Study Group. N Engl J Med. 1992;326(17):1123–9.

10. Patwa HS, Chaudhry V, Katzberg H, Rae-Grant AD, So YT. Evidence-based guideline: intravenous immunoglobulin in the treatment of neuromuscular disorders: report of the Therapeutics and Technology Assessment Subcommittee of the American Academy of Neurology. Neurology. 2012;78(13):1009–15.

11. Randomised trial of plasma exchange, intravenous immunoglobulin, and combined treatments in Guillain-Barré syndrome. Plasma Exchange/Sandoglobulin Guillain-Barré Syndrome Trial Group. Lancet. 1997;349(9047):225–30.

Hypoxic ischemic brain injury

Mypinder S. Sekhon and Donald E. Griesdale

Ischemic injury to cerebral tissue is secondary to generalized decreased cerebral oxygen delivery from cardiac arrest secondary to VT/VF or PEA.

Etiology

Table 14.1 Etiology of cardiac arrest

Category	Specific etiology		
Ventricular tachycardia	Monomorphic	Structurally normal heart	RVOT Idiopathic VT
		Structurally abnormal heart	Previous CAD/scar tissue Cardiomyopathy, HOCM ARVD
	Polymorphic	Dilated cardiomyopathy Ischemia Prolonged QT Brugada syndrome	
Ventricular fibrillation	Usually degenerative rhythm from ventricular tachycardia		
Pulseless electrical activity	Hypoxia Hypothermia Hypoglycemia Hyperkalemia Hypovolemia H⁺ – Acidosis		Thrombosis – PE/MI Tension pneumothorax Trauma Toxins Tamponade

RVOT = Right ventricular outflow tachycardia, VT = Ventricular tachycardia, CAD = Coronary artery disease, ARVD = Arrhythmogenic right ventricular dysplasia, PE = Pulmonary embolism, MI = Myocardial infarction, HOCM = Hypertrophic obstructive cardiomyopathy.

Diagnosis

Table 14.2 States of altered conciousness

Condition	Awareness	Arousal	Sleep–wake cycles	Motor
Persistent vegetative	No	Yes	Yes	Non-purposeful
Minimally conscious	No	Yes	Yes	Occasionally purposeful
Akinetic mutism	No	Yes	Yes	No
Locked-in state	Yes	Yes	Yes	Vertical eye movement
Coma	No	No	No	Non-purposeful
Brain death	No	No	No	No

(Adapted from *Crit Care Med, 2006; 31:31–42.*)

The brain is a highly metabolically active organ which requires up to 20% of the cardiac output for normal functioning. After a cardiac arrest and cessation of cerebral blood flow, neuronal ischemia can result in permanent infarction within minutes. Gray matter and deeper brain structures such as the basal ganglia are especially vulnerable to ischemic insults.

Neurologic determination of death

Pre-conditions
1. Diagnosis of condition with the potential for irreversible brain injury
2. Exclusion of confounders
a) Central nervous system depressant medications
b) Hypothermia (central temperature < 35°C)
c) Metabolic/Cardiorespiratory / Endocrine disturbance

Clinical Exam	
Clinical Finding	**Conditions**
Brain Stem reflexes	
a) Pupil	Pupils mid or dilated position, fixed, no response bilaterally to light stimulus
b) Corneal	No response to cotton stimuli to cornea
c) Gag	No response to posterior pharyngeal wall
d) Cough	No response to tracheal suction
e) Oculo-cephalic	Iris fixed in mid-position with axial rotation of ñeck
f) Vestibulo-ocular	Iris fixed in mid-position with cold stimuli to external auditory canals bilaterally
Motor Examination	No response to noxious stimuli (excluding spinal reflexes)

Apnea Testing

Apnea test

Condtitions
1. Pre-oxygenate patient with 100% FiO_2 for 5 minutes
2. Arterial blood gas to confirm normal pH and initial pCO_2
3. Cease ventilation and maintain administration of 100% FiO_2 with a closed system CPAP between for 8–10 cmH_2O
4. Observe patiennt for respiration
5. Repeat arterial blood gas to confirm pCO_2 rise > 20 mmHg and pH < 7_30 without respiratory efforts observed

If all conditions not met:
Ancillary testing required:
1. Four vessel angiogram
2. Cerebral scientigraphy

If all conditions not met:
BRAIN DEATH

Figure 14.1 Diagnostic approach to clinical brain death.

Anoxic brain injury

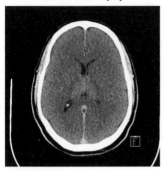

1) Absence of grey–white differentiation
2) Appearance of basal ganglia obscured
3) Sulci compressed indicates cerebral edema

Normal CT head

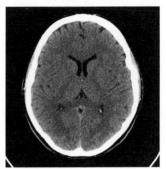

1) Presence of grey–white differentiation
2) Appearance of basal ganglia intact
3) Sulci present

Figure 14.2 Computed tomography of normal vs. anoxic–ischemic brain injury. CT evidence of anoxic brain injury includes grey–white differentiation loss and obliteration of the basal ganglia as these are especially predisposed to anoxia due to high oxygen uptake and metabolism. Absence of sulci indicates diffuse cerebral edema after anoxia.

Management

Table 14.3 Management approach to anoxic–ischemic brain injury

Approach	Intervention
Evaluate and treat underlying cause	VT/VF a. Echocardiogram b. Coronary angiogram c. Electrophysiology study d. MRI (for ARVD) ICD for post VT/VF
Hypothermia	Indication criteria a. VT/VF arrest b. Timing > 10 min and < 60 min until ROSC c. GCS < 10 d. Stable hemodynamics e. Age > 18

Table 14.3 (cont.)

Approach	Intervention
	Contraindications a. Coagulopathy (Plts < 30, INR > 2.5) b. Recurrent VT/VF or unstable arrhythmias c. Refractory shock/hypotension despite vasopressors + fluids d. Actively bleeding (esp. intracranial hemorrhage) Hypothermia management a. Sedation and mechanical ventilation b. Temperature goal: 35–36°C × 72 h. Strictly avoid hyperthermia c. Neuromuscular blockade prn for shivering d. MAP goal 70–80 mmHg with vasopressor support Hypothermia complications a. Arrhythmias – recurrent VT, bradyarrythmias, prolonged QT b. Electrolyte disturbance (hypokalemia) c. Bleeding risk d. Infection e. Glucose disturbances, ileus
Complications	Status epilepticus – apply status epilepticus protocol Cerebral edema – apply TBI increased ICP protocol

VT = Ventricular tachycardia, VF = Ventricular fibrillation, ARVD = Arrhythmogenic right ventricular dysplasia, ICD = Implantable cardioverter defibrillator, MRI = Magnetic resonance imaging, ROSC = Return of spontaneous circulation, MAP = Mean arterial pressure, ICP = Intracranial pressure.

Prognosis

Exclude confounders

a. Central nervous system depressant medications
b. Hypothermia (central temperature < 35°C)
c. Metabolic/cardiorespiratory/endocrine disturbance

Table 14.4 Neurologic prognosis of anoxic–ischemic brain injury – hypothermia vs. normothermia

Hypothermia			Normothermia		
Day	Prognosticator	Outcome	Day	Prognosticator	Outcome
1	Myoclonic status epilepticus	Poor	1	Myoclonic status epilepticus	Poor
1–3	NSE > 33 ng/ml	Unclear	1–3	NSE > 33 umol/l	Poor
1–3	Absence of N_2O on SSEP	Poor	1–3	Absence of N_2O on SSEP	Poor
3	Absence of motor or decerebrate	Unclear	3	Absence of motor or decerebrate	Poor
3	Absence of pupil/corneal reflexes	Poor	3	Absence of pupil/corneal reflexes	Poor

SSEP = Somatosensory evoked potentials, NSE = Neuron-specific enolase.

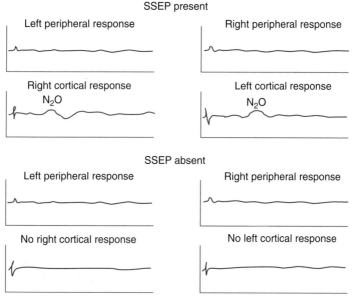

Figure 14.3 Comparison of presence and absence of N_2O response. The absence of the N_2O response portends a poor neurological outcome in post cardiac arrest patients.

Table 14.5 Somatosensory evoked potentials

Overview	Somatosensory evoked potentials result from stimuli to the peripheral nerves (median nerve most common for post cardiac arrest). The electrical impulse is carried to the primary somatosoensory cortex from the peripheral nerves, spinal cord dorsal columns, brainstem, thalamocortical projections and finally to the cortex. The latency of the N_2O response is used in the prognostication of cardiac arrest.
Acquisition	An electrode is placed over the median nerve and receiving electrodes are placed on the scalp. An electrical impulse is initiated at the median nerve and the latency of the transmission of the electrial impulse is measured at the scalp/somatosensory cortex.
Result interpretation	Bilateral absence of the N_2O response portends a poor prognosis in anoxic– ischemic brain injury. Abnormalities in SSEP response can be secondary to damage in the peripheral nerves, plexus, spinal cord, brainstem, thalami or cortex.
Pitfalls	Coma complicated by metabolic or infectious factors can make the result potentially unreliable.

Evidence-based neurocritical care

Table 14.6 The role of hypothermia in anoxic brain injury

Question	Use of hypothermia in post cardiac arrest anoxic brain injury
Summary	Two previous trials demonstrated an improved neurologic outcome in patients with an out of hospital cardiac arrest due to non-perfusion ventricular arrthymias. However, these trials were criticized, in part due to permissive hyperthermia in the control arms. A recent trial randomized 950 patients who were unconcious following an out-of-hospital cardiac arrest to 33°C vs. 36°C. There was no difference in patients who had a poor neurologic outcome (54% vs. 52%) at 180 days. A strength of the trial was the protocolized method for withdrawal of life-sustaining therapy.

Summary

- Anoxic brain injury is the result of insufficient global cerebral oxygen delivery, which results in diffuse cerebral ischemia and infarction.
- The diagnosis of anoxic brain injury encompasses detailed history and clinical examination. Imaging studies may support the diagnosis but are insufficient in isolation for diagnosis or prognostication.
- The management of anoxic brain injury involves therapeutic hypothermia (if VT/VF) and adequate cerebral oxygen delivery to help support the injured brain.

- Prognostication requires an accurate clinical exam with use of supportive tests such as somatosensory evoked potentials and biomarkers.
- Brain death declaration is a complex process requiring a detailed clinical examination, apnea testing and an appropriate accompanying clinical history. In the setting of an ambiguous clinical examination, ancillary imaging testing can be completed.

Suggested readings

1. The Hypothermia after Cardiac Arrest Study Group. Mild therapeutic hypothermia to improve the neurologic outcome after cardiac arrest. N Engl J Med. 2002;346:549–556.

2. Young BG. Neurologic prognosis after cardiac arrest. NEJM. 2009;361:(6): 605–611.

3. Fugate JE, Wijdicks E, Mandrekar J, et al. Predictors of neurological outcome in hypothermia after cardiac arrest. Ann Neurol. 2010;68:907–914.

4. Wijdicks E, Hijdra A, Young BG, et al. Practice parameter: Prediction of outcome in comatose survivors after cardiopulmonary resuscitation (an evidence-based review): Report of the Quality Standards Subcommittee of the American Association of Neurology. Neurology. 2006;76:203–210.

5. Shemie SD, Baker AJ, Knoll G, Wall W, Rocker G, Howes D, et al. National recommendations for donation after cardiocirculatory death in Canada: Donation after cardiocirculatory death in Canada. CMAJ. 2006 Oct 10;175(8):S1.

6. Bernard SA, Gray TW, Buist MD, et al. Treatment of comatose survivors of out-of-hospital cardiac arrest with induced hypothermia. N Engl J Med. 2002;346(8):557–563.

7. Nielsen N, Wetterslev J, Cronberg T, et al. Targeted temperature management at 33°C versus 36°C after cardiac arrest. N Engl J Med. 2013;369(23):2197–2206.

Chapter 15

Central nervous system infections

Indeep S. Sekhon and Mypinder S. Sekhon

Meningitis is an infection of the meningeal membranes and subarachnoid space by a microbe.

Encephalitis is an infection of the cerebral parenchyma by a microbe resulting in impaired cortical and/or subcortical function.

Etiology and diagnosis

Table 15.1 Bacterial meningitis etiology

Microbe	Incidence	Risk factors
S. pneumoniae	30–60%	Disseminated *S. pneumoniae*, upper resp. infection
N. meningiditis	10–35%	Young adults, close contacts, complement deficiencies
H. influenzae	< 5%	Preceding upper respiratory tract infection
L. monocytogenes	5–10%	Immunocompromised, elderly, alcoholics, hemochromatosis
S. aureus	5%	Recent neurosurgical procedure/head trauma
Gram-negative	1–0%	Nosocomial, concurrent gastrointestinal helminth infection

Table 15.2 Aseptic meningitis etiology

Category	Causes	Cerebrospinal fluid analysis
Infection	Viral a. Enteroviruses b. Herpes viruses (HSV) c. Other – HIV, LCMV, mumps	Lymphocyte predominance Exceptions: a. Early enterovirus = PMNs b. LCMV = occ. low glucose and WBCs > 1,000
	Bacterial a. Partially treated bacterial meningitis b. Mycobacterium – TB c. Spirochetal – treponema, borrelia	Lymphocyte predominance Early TB – high PMNs, low glucose Late TB – increased lymphocytes
	Fungal a. Cryptococcus b. Coccidiomycosis c. Tick borne d. Rickettsia e. Ehrlichiosis	Crypto = monocyte predominance, low glucose Coccidio = increased esoinophils Lymphocyte predominance
Medications	Sulfa drugs, NSAIDs, isoniazid IVIG, anticonvulsants	Mild PMN predominance
Malignancy	Leptomeningeal spread a. Intracranial tumors b. Carcinomatous meningitis c. Lymphoma	Lymphocyte predominance Hodgkin lymphoma a. Increased eosinophils
Inflammatory	Behçet's Systemic lupus eythematosis Sarcoidosis	Lymphocyte predominance

HSV = Herpes simplex virus, HIV = Human immunodeficiency virus, LCMV = Lymphocytic choriomeningitis virus, TB = Tuberculosis, PMN = Polymorphionuclear neutrophils, WBC = White blood count, NSAID = Non-steroidal anti-inflammatory drugs, IVIG = Intravenous immunoglobulin.

Table 15.3 Enchephalitis etiology

Category		Microbiology	MRI pattern
Infectious	Viral	Enteroviruses Herpes viruses Arboviruses Other – HIV, rabies	Non-specific LE Thalami, BG, LE Non-specific
	Bacterial	*L. monocytogenes* *M. tuberculosis*	RE RE

Table 15.3 (cont.)

Category		Antibody	Associations	MRI pattern
Antibody-mediated	Paraneoplastic	Anti-NMDA	Ovarian teratoma	LE or normal
		Anti-Hu	Lung, neuroblastoma	LE, RE, DE
		Anti-Ma2	Testicular, lung, breast	LE, RE, DE
		Anti-CASPR2	Thymus, uterine	LE
		Anti CRMP5	Lung, thymus	LE, CE, SE
		Anti-LGI1	Lung, thyroid, renal, thymus	LE, normal
		Anti-GABA$_B$	Lung	LE, normal
		Anti-AMPAR	Lung, breast	LE
		Anti-Yo	Ovarian, breast, uterine	CE
		Anti-Ri	Ovarian, breast, lung	RE, CE
	Autoimmune	Anti-VGKC	Autoimmune	LE
		Anti-NMO	Neuromyelitis optica	RE, optic nerve

LE = Limbic encephalitis, RE= Rhomboencephalitis, DE = Diencephalon encephalitis, CE = Cerebellar encephalitis, SE = Striatal encephalitis, BG = Basal ganglia, NMO = Neuromyelitis optica, VGKC = Voltage-gated potassium channel.

Complications

Table 15.4 Complications of meningitis

Complication	Therapy
Cerebral edema	Treat underlying cause Apply TBI protocol approach to increased ICP
Status epilepticus	Treat underlying cause Apply status epilepticus protocol
Intracranial hemorrhage	Treat underlying cause Apply intracranial hemorrhage protocol
Cerebral venous thrombosis	Require definitive imaging diagnosis (CT or MR venogram) Treatment = anticoagulation – intravenous UFH
Ischemic stroke	Exclude other causes of ischemic stroke Supportive management
Cranial subdural empyema	Broad-spectrum antibiotics Surgical drainage
Intracranial abscess	Broad-spectrum antibiotics Surgical drainage if > 2.5 cm

ICP = Intracranial pressure, CT = Computed tomography, MR = Magnetic resonance, UFH = Unfractionated heparin.

Table 15.5 Bacterial abscess

Epidemiology	Incidence 1:10,000 hospitalized patients in developed world	
Risk factors	Contiguous spread from alternative infection site Male gender Immunocompromised Recent neurosurgical procedure or open skull fracture	
Microbiology	Immunocompetent host	Polymicrobial in 60% of all cases. Microbiology depends on source of contiguous site of infection
		Oral/upper resp: source: streptococci, fusobacterium, prevotella, bacteroides (not *B. frag.*)
		Paranasal sinus: staph., enterobacter
		Ear: pseudomonas, staph., strep.
		Post surgical: staph., Gram-negative rods
	Immunocompromised host	Bacterial: All of the above, *Listeria m.* Fungal: histoplasma, blastomycosis, coccidiomycosis, cryptococcus, aspergillus, nocardia
Pathogenesis	Direct spread from contiguous infection site occurs in 50% of cases. Intracranial spread occurs from adjacent bony infection, bacterial invasion of emissary veins of skull or via lymphatics Most common sites are: a. Paranasal sinuses – frontal/temporal lobes b. Middle ear infections – temporal lobe/cerebellum c. Dental abscesses – frontal lobe d. Deep tissue neck infections – frontal lobe e. Mastoiditis – temporal lobe/cerebellum Hematogenous spread – most commonly from bacterial endocarditis or endovascular infection. Accounts for 25% of brain abscesses Meningitis rarely accounts for brain abscess Rare associations: Osler Weber Rendu, Klebsiella brain abscess with concomitant liver abscesses, cyanotic heart disease Stages of brain abscess formation: a. Day 1–3: Direct cerebritis from bacterial infection/innoculation b. Day 4–9: Cerebritis expands and necrotic center develops c. Day 10–14: Capsule formation which is vascularized. Ring enhancing lesion on CT	
Diagnosis	Clinical: Headache, altered LOC, seizures, focal neurological deficit, meningeal signs Microbiology: Blood, CSF and tissue cultures of adjacent infection site (if possible) Imaging: Computed tomography with and without contrast. Consider MRI with angiography if CT images do not provide adequate tissue detail Lumbar puncture should be performed if no contraindications	

Table 15.5 (cont.)

Imaging	Computed tomography with contrast. Appearance of malignancy can be difficult as many are also ring enhancing on CT with contrast. Brain abscesses have a "smooth" rim appearance as opposed to an irregular rim with maligancies
	MRI with contrast. Advantage includes greater sensitivity and also can detect adjacent cerebritis with abscess
	Appearance of multiple abscesses indicates likely hematogenous source
Treatment	Evaluate for primary infection site. If identified, source control should be achieved
	Medical: Initial therapy should target Gram-positives (staph. and strep.), Gram-negatives and anaerobes. If cultures are not obtained with a culprit organism, continue empiric antimicrobials for 6–8 weeks targeting Gram positives/negatives and upper airway anaerobes
	Reassessment of therapy: CT every 2 weeks to assess efficacy of antimicrobial therapy
	Abx with CNS penetration: Ceftriaxone/meropenem/metronidazole/penicillin G
	Surgical: Abscesses > 2.5 cm: stereotactic aspiration/drainage or excision

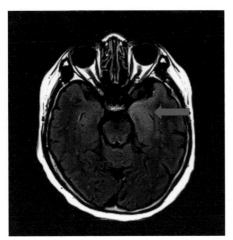

Figure 15.1 Magnetic resonance imaging demonstrating herpes simplex virus limbic encephalitis. Temporal lobar hemorrhage typically ensues after HSV infection of the cerebral parenchyma.

Management

Table 15.6 Antimicrobial management in meningitis

Category	Disease	Therapy
Viral	HSV/VZV	Acyclovir 10 mg/kg IV every 8 hours
	CMV	Gancyclovir + Foscarnet
	HHV-6	Gancyclovir or Foscarnet
	HIV	ARVs
	Arboviruses	Interferon 2 alpha
	Measles	Ribavirin
	All others	Supportive
Bacterial	Community acquired	Regimens a. Ceftriaxone + vancomycin b. Meropenem + vancomycin (β-lactam allergy) Corticosteroids a. Dexamethasone – start prior or with antibiotics for *S. pneumo.* & GCS 8–11 Prophylaxis – for *N. meningitis*, a. Ciprofloxacin 500 mg × 1 b. Rifampin 600 mg BID × 2 days c. Ceftriaxone 250 mg IM × 1 Isolation – droplet precautions until Abx × 24h
	Nosocomial	Regimens a. Meropenem + vancomycin b. Ceftazidime + vancomycin
	Immunocompromised	Regimens a. Ceftriaxone + vancomycin + ampicillin TB – quadruple therapy + dexamethasone
Fungal	Cryptococcus	Induction: amphotericin + 5-flucytosine × 2 weeks Consolidation: high-dose fluconazole × 4 weeks Maintenance/prophylaxis: fluconazole × 10 weeks Therapeutic lumbar puncture a. Decrease opening by 50% if greater than 40 cm b. Decrease opening pressure to < 20 cm if initial < 40

HSV = Herpes simplex virus, CMV = Cytomegalovirus, HHV = Human herpes virus, HIV = Human immunodeficiency virus ARV = Anti retroviral, VZV = Varicella Zoster virus.

Table 15.7 Diagnosis and management of nosocomial ventriculitis

Category	Details
Risk factors	a) EVD in situ b) EVD duration > 5–7 days c) Hemorrhagic CSF d) Frequent routine CSF sampling e) Aseptic technique of CSF sampling
Microbiology	Gram-positives – 75% a) *Staphylococcus epideridis* b) *Staphylococcus Aureus* Gram-negatives – 25% a) *E. coli* b) Enterobacter c) Pseudomonas d) Klebsiella e) Acinetobacter

Diagnosis	a) Organism cultured from CSF
	b) Patient has at least one of:
	   1) Fever (> 38°C)
	   2) Altered mental status
	   3) Headache
	   4) Stiff neck
	   5) Meningeal signs
	   6) Cranial nerve palsies
	
	And one of:
	   1) Increased CSF WBCs, protein, decreased glucose
	   2) Gram stain positive for organisms
	   3) Organisms cultured from blood
	   4) CSF, blood, urine antigen positive for microbe

Treatment	Antimicrobial therapy a) Meropenem (2g IV q8h) + vancomycin b) Ceftazidime + vancomycin Consideration of EVD removal/replacement Intrathecal antibiotics (vancomycin and aminoglycosides) Duration of therapy should be dictated on a case by case basis Minimum duration 10–14 days

Evidence-based neurocritical care

Table 15.8 Role of steroids in meningitis

Question	The role of steroids as adjunctive therapy in bacterial meningitis
Summary	In this trial 301 patients with acute bacterial meningitis were randomized to adjuvant dexamethasone (10 mg IV prior to antibiotics, then every 6 hours for 4 days) vs. placebo. Patients receiving dexamethasone had reduced risk of an unfavourable outcome (RR 0.59, 95% CI 0.37 to 0.94, p = 0.03). This risk reduction was observed in the subgroup of patients with meningitis secondary to *Streptococcal pneumoniae*. It also appears that these benefits are only observed with dexamethasone if administered prior to the patient receiving antibiotics.

Summary

- Central nervous system infections can lead to devastating long-term neurological sequelae.
- Prompt diagnosis and management with antimicrobials is of paramount importance to improve outcomes. If possible, imaging and cerebrospinal fluid analysis with lumbar puncture should be completed.
- Complications of CNS infections are common and may require surgical therapy and advanced critical care management.
- Cerebral abscess is a life-threatening condition which results from numerous microbes. Contrast imaging and potential aspiration are required for diagnosis. Treatment consists of antimicrobial therapy and surgical drainage in severe cases.

Suggested readings

1. Beckman JD, Tyler K. Neurointensive care of patients with acute CNS infections. Neurotherapeutics. 2011;1:1–15.

2. Schut E, Lucas MJ, Brouwer MC et al. Cerebral infarction in adults with bacterial meningitis. Neurocrit Care. 2011;3:943–950.

3. Ziai WC, Lewin JJ 3rd. Update in the diagnosis and management of central nervous system infections. Neurol Clin. 2008 May;26(2):427–468.

4. Beer R, Lackner P, Pfausler B, Schmutzhard E. Nosocomial ventriculitis and meningitis in neurocritical care patients. J Neurol. 2008 Nov;255(11):1617–1624.

5. Beer R, Pfausler B, Schmutzhard E. Infectious intracranial complications in the neuro-ICU patient population. Curr Opin Crit Care. 2010 Apr;16(2):117–122.

6. De Gans J, van de Beek D. Dexamethasone in adults with bacterial meningitis. N Engl J Med. 2002;347(20):1549–1556.

Chapter 16

Cerebral venous sinus thrombosis

Indeep S. Sekhon and Mypinder S. Sekhon

Definition: Thrombosis in the cerebral venous vasculature resulting in clot formation.

Epidemiology: 3:1 female ratio: 60–75% of patients have a good functional outcome.

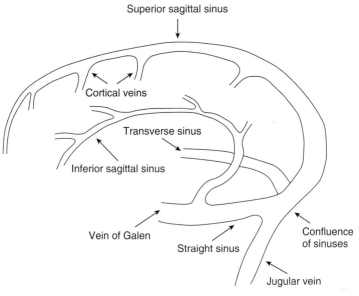

Figure 16.1 Cerebral venous sinus anatomy. Cortical veins drain into both superior and inferior sagittal venous sinuses. The transverse and sigmoid sinuses provide venous drainage from the inferior aspects of the frontal, parietal, occipital and temporal lobes. The vein of Galen drains the deep cerebral structures and forms the straight sinus once joined by the inferior sagittal sinus. Ultimately, all sinuses converge at the confluence of sinuses which leads into the internal jugular veins.

Table 16.1 Etiology of hypercoaguable states resulting in cerebral venous sinus thrombosis

Category	Etiology	Clinical pearls/diagnosis
Congenital	Factor V Leiden	Concomitant smoking – higher risk
	Prothrombin mutation	G20210A mutation leads to increased prothrombin levels
	Protein C or S deficiency	Cannot test if active clot or anticoagulation
	ATIII deficiency	Cannot test if active clot or anticoagulation
	Antiphospholipid syndrome	Associated with SLE
Acquired	Malignancy	Carcinomas – highest risk
	Hormonal	Post partum – highest risk, 1:10,000 births
	a. Pregnancy	Higher risk with concurrent smoking
	b. Estrogen-based OCP	
	c. Estrogen-based HRT	
	Nephrotic syndrome	Hypercoaguable because ATIII, protein C/S deficiency from renal losses
	Platelet disorders – HIT	Isolated cerebral thrombosis rare
	Trauma	Usually clot in adjacent sinus to focal injury
	Infectious	Meningitis or encephalitis
	Paroxysmal nocturnal hemoglobinuria	Concomitant mesenteric venous clots
		Associated cytopenias and leukemic transformation

Table 16.2 Diagnostic work-up for cerebral sinus thrombosis and underlying thrombophilias

	Investigations	Specifics
Imaging	CT head	Multiple hemorrhages located diffusely in lobar distribution
		Focal cerebral edema – region of single venous sinus drainage
		Dense clot sign in confluence of sinuses
	CT venogram	Sensitivity ~ 90%, specificity ~ 95%
	MR venogram	Sensitivity > 95%, specificity > 95%
	Venogram	Gold standard examination but 2% complication rate
Thrombophilia	Factor V Leiden	PCR test
	Prothrombin gene	PCR test
	Antiphospholipid Abs	Lupus anticoagulant, anti-cardiolipin Ab, anti-B2 microglobulin Ab

Table 16.2 (cont.)

Investigations	Specifics
Protein C/S deficiency	Protein C/S deficiency measured with functional assay, therefore not accurate in setting of acute clot or systemic anticoagulation
ATIII deficiency	Anithrombin III deficiency measured with functional assay, therefore not accurate in setting of acute clot or systemic anticoagulation
Secondary cause	Evaluate for underlying malignancy, hormonal causes, nephrotic syndrome or concurrent CNS infection
	PNH – peripheral flow cytometry for CD 55 and CD 59

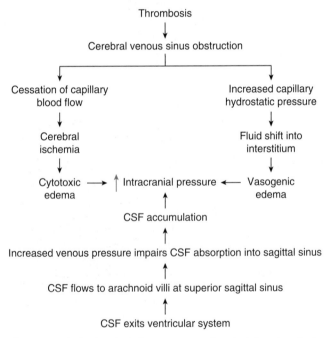

Figure 16.2 Pathophysiological consequences of cerebral sinus thrombosis.

CT non-contrast showing cortical microhemorrhages

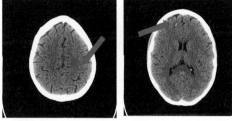

Figure 16.3 Computed tomography non-contrast and venogram evidence of cerebral venous sinus thrombosis. Multiple punctate hemorrhages in a single venous distribution located diffusely throughout the cerebral parenchyma is a sign on CT to suggest underlying cerebral venous sinus thrombosis. This finding should warrant prompt CT venography.

Evidence of superior sagittal venous sinus thrombosis

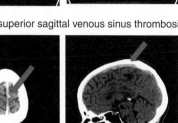

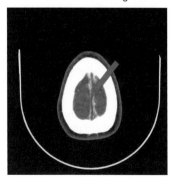

CT venogram with evidence of thrombosis

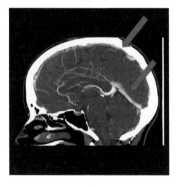

Figure 16.4 CT venogram evidence of cerebral venous sinus thrombosis. This CT venogram demonstrates a filling defect in the superior sagittal sinus. This is the most common location of thrombosis.

Evaluate and treat underlying cause/precipitant	
Anticoagulation	**Comments**
Unfractionated heparin & LMWH	Systemic anticoagulation has been evaluated in 3 RCTs and a pooled meta-analysis shows a non-statistically significant reduction in death/dependency. Expert opinion advises to commence heparin-based anticoagulation in cerebral venous sinus thrombosis, even in the presence of hemorrhage.
Thrombin inhibitors	No evidence/role
Factor X inhibitors	No evidence/role
Anti-platelets	No evidence/role
Vitamin K antagonists	Bridge to vitamin K antagonists (coumadin) over 48–72 h with therapeutic anticoagulation with heparin. Use VKAs for long-term anticoagulation over 6 months, if not longer, depending on underlying disease entity/precipitant.
Thrombolysis — Systemic	No evidence/role
Thrombolysis — Catheter directed	Evidence for endovascular venous administration of thombolysis is limited to case series. Often combined with catheter-based clot extraction.

Summary

- Cerebral venous sinus thrombosis occurs as a result of underlying inherited thombophilias or acquired hypercoaguability states.
- Thrombosis in the cerebral venous sinuses can lead to hemorrhage, vasogenic cerebral edema and obstruction of CSF absorption, all of which can produce increased ICP.
- Diagnosis requires careful history and examination for predisposing conditions and imaging. Non-contrast CT may reveal intraparenchymal hemorrhage and a venogram/venography will yield the presence of a filling defect in the cerebral venous vasculature.
- Management focuses on treating the underlying cause, systemic anticoagulation with heparin-based products and potentially endovascular techniques using clot extraction/thrombolysis.

Suggested readings

1. Stam J. Thrombosis of the cerebral veins and sinuses. NEJM. 2005; 352: 1791–1798.

2. Bousser MG, Ross-Russell RW. *Cerebral Venous Sinus Thrombosis*. London. WB Saunders. 1997.

3. Lanska DJ, Kryscio RJ. Risk factors for peripartum and postpartum stroke and intracranial venous thrombosis. Stroke. 2000; 31: 1274.

4. Saposnik G, Barinagarrementeria F, Brown RD Jr, et al. Diagnosis and management of cerebral venous thrombosis: a statement for healthcare professionals from the American Heart Association/American Stroke Association. Stroke. 2011; 42: 1158.

Cerebral vasculitis

Mypinder S. Sekhon

Definition: Inflammatory infiltrate involving the cerebral vascular vessels resulting in neurological dysfunction and ischemia.

Table 17.1 Approach to CNS vasculitis

Category	Description	
Primary	Isolated vasculitis of the central nervous system (brain and spinal cord) No systemic manifestations Require a biopsy for definitive diagnosis	
Secondary	Autoimmune	**Large wall** Takayasu's arteritis Giant cell arteritis **Medium wall** Polyarteritis nodosa Kawasaki's **Small wall** ANCA associated a. Wegener's granulomatosis b. Churg–Strauss c. Microscopic polyangiitis Immune complex-mediated a. Connective tissue associated (SLE, RA) b. Cryoglobulinemia c. Behçet's d. Henoch–Schönlein purpura Miscellaneous a. Sarcoidosis
	Paraneoplastic	Lymphatoid granulomatosis Intravascular lymphoma

Table 17.1 (cont.)

Category	Description	
	Drug induced	Amphetamines
		Ephedrine
		Methylphenidate
	Infectious	Varicella zoster virus
		Human immunodeficiency virus
		Cytomegalovirus
		Parvovirus B19
		Treponema pallidum

Table 17.2 Clinical features of systemic vasculidities and CNS/organ manifestations

Name	Nervous system involvement	Organ involvement	Serology/ associations
		Large	
Takayasu's arteritis	TIA, ischemic embolic stroke from cranial aortic branch stenosis	Aorta & major aortic branches	Young females Asian descent
GCA	Headache	Temporal arteritis Constitutional Sx Optic neuritis/ amaurosis fugax	Polymyalgia rheumatica
		Medium	
PAN	Mononeuritis multiplex	Renal – GN, AKI, HTN GI – mesenteric ischemia & aneurysms Skin – livedo reticularis, purpura, Testicular pain	Hep B p-ANCA ~ 20%
		Small – ANCA	
Wegener's	Aseptic meningitis Cerebral vasculitis – rare Mononeuritis multiplex	Renal – GN Pulmonary – nodules, hemorrhage Upper airway – nasal, ears, sinuses Ocular – uevitis, episcleritis	c-ANCA – 90%

Table 17.2 (cont.)

Name	Nervous system involvement	Organ involvement	Serology/ associations
Churg– Strauss	CNS involvement – 5% of cases Mononeuritis multiplex	Renal – GN Pulmonary – asthma, fleeting infiltrates Cardiac – arteritis/ myocarditis Heme – eosinophilia	p-ANCA – 50%
MPA	CNS involvement – 5% of cases Mononeuritis multiplex	Renal – GN Pulmonary – capillaritis, hemorrhage	p-ANCA – 70%
		Small – Immune complex	
RA	Cerebral vasculitis/ cerebritis	Joint – synovitis Pulmonary – effusions, fibrosis Cardiac	RF Anti-CCP Seronegative – 5%
SLE	Cerebral vasculitis/ cerebritis Psychosis Seizures Cerebral venous thrombosis	Rash – photosensitivity, discoid, malar Renal – GN, nephrotic syndrome Joint –non-erosive arthritis Hemolysis, thrombocytopenia Pulmonary – hemorrhage, HTN Serositis – cardiac, pulmonary	ANA, Anti-dsDNA Anti-Smith Anti-La, Anti-Ro Antiphospholipid Ab
CG	Mononeuritis multiplex Peripheral neuropathy	Renal – GN Skin – livedo reticularis, purpura Arthralgias	Cryocrit, RF Hep C
Behçet's	CNS manifestations – 30% Cerebral venous thrombosis Meningoencephalitis Rhomboencephalitis	Skin – mucosal ulcers Genital – ulcers Joint – arthritis	Pathergy test (poor sens. & spec.)

Table 17.2 (cont.)

Name	Nervous system involvement	Organ involvement	Serology/ associations
		Miscellaneous	
Sarcoid	Aseptic meningitis Cerebral vasculitis/ cerebritis Granulomatous infiltration of brainstem	Joint Pulmonary – fibrosis, pulm. HTN Cardiac – RCMP, conduction Dx	Hypercalcemia Serum ACE + (poor sens. & spec.)

CNS = Central nervous system, GCA = Giant cell arteritis, PAN = Polyarteritis nodosa, MPA = Microscopic polyangiitis, RA = Rheumatoid arthritis, SLE = Systemic lupus erythematosis, CG = Cryoglobulinemia.

Table 17.3 Diagnosis and treatment of systemic vasculidties affecting the CNS

Name	Diagnosis	Treatment
		Large
Takayasu's	a. Age < 40 b. Claudication c. Bruits d. Extremity BP diff > 10 mmHg e. Arteritis on angiogram f. Dec brachial artery pulse	Corticosteroids (prednisone 1 mg/kg) Methotrexate
GCA	a. Age > 50 b. Headache c. ESR > 50 d. Temporal artery biopsy e. Temporal artery tenderness	Corticosteroids (prednisone 1 mg/kg/d)
		Medium
PAN	a. Weight loss > 4 kg b. Livedo reticularis c. Myalgia d. Hep B +	Corticosteroids Cyclophosphamide Anti-Hep B Tx (if Hep B active assoc. PAN)

Table 17.3 (cont.)

Name	Diagnosis	Treatment
	e. Neuropathy f. Diastolic BP > 90 mmHg g. Cr > 150 h. Biopsy positive i. Angio abnormal j. Testicular pain/ tenderness	

	Small – ANCA	
Wegener's	a. Nasal or oral inflammation b. Lung cavities, nodules, infiltrates c. Microscopic hematuria, RBC casts d. Granulomatous infiltration on biopsy	Corticosteroids –1 g/d × 3d then Pred 1 mg/kg (for pulm. hemorrhage, CNS vasculitis, anuric renal disease) Cyclophosphamide Plasmapheresis (Pulm. Hemo., CNS Dx)
Churg–Strauss	a. Asthma b. Eosinophilia c. Neuropathy d. Pulmonary infiltrates e. Paranasal sinus abnormality f. Extravascular eosinophils on biopsy	Corticosteroids – 1 g/d × 3d then Pred. 1 mg/kg (for pulm. hemorrhage, CNS vasculitis, anuric renal disease) Cyclophosphamide Plasmapheresis (Pulm. Hemo., CNS Dx)
MPA	a. Biopsy – necrotizing, non-granulomatous b. p-ANCA + c. Does not meet criteria for WG or CS	Corticosteroids – 1 g/d × 3d then Pred 1 mg/kg (for pulm. hemorrhage, CNS vasculitis, anuric renal disease) Cyclophosphamide Plasmapheresis (Pulm. hemo., CNS Dx)

	Small – Immune complex	
RA	a. AM stiffness b. Hand arthritis c. Rheumatoid nodules d. X-rays with erosive arthritis changes e. Symmetric joint arthritis f. Arthritis > 3 joints g. + RF	Corticosteroids Cyclophosphamide for CNS Dx

Table 17.3 (cont.)

Name	Diagnosis	Treatment
SLE	a. Malar rash b. Discoid rash c. Photosensitivity d. Arthritis e. Serositis f. Psychosis or seizures g. Proteinuria/RBC casts h. Oral ulcers i. Hemolysis, low plts j. + ANA h. Anti-dsDNA, Anti-Smith	Cerebral vascultis assoc. SLE a. Pulse corticosteroids b. Cyclophosphamide c. Anti–TNF therapy
CG	a. + Cryocrit b. + Cryoglobulin electrophoresis c. + Rheumatoid factor d. + Hep C serology e. Decreased C4, normal C3	Treat underlying cause a. Lymphoproliferative Dx b. Hep C c. Underlying infection corticosteroids, plasmapheresis
Behçet's	a. Genital ulcers b. Oral ulcers c. Pathergy + d. Pustules, erythema nodosum e. Eyes – uveitis, episcleritis, optic neuritis	Corticosteroids +/– cyclophosphamide for CNS manifestations Azathioprine for ocular Dx & ulcerations
Miscellaneous		
Sarcoidosis	Biopsy with non-caseating granulomas	Corticosteroids

Summary

- Cerebral vasculitis is a state of inflammation in the cerebral vasculature resulting in ischemia and neurological dysfunction.
- The etiology of cerebral vasculitis is most commonly secondary to a systemic disorder; however, primary cerebral vasculitis is increasingly becoming recognized.

- Diagnosis requires a careful history/examination for associated conditions. Cerebral imaging can identify abnormal appearance of the cerebral vasculature consistent with vasculitis.
- Management depends on the underlying cause of cerebral vasculitis.

Suggested readings

1. Calabrese LH, Duna GF, Lie JT. Vasculitis in the central nervous system. Arthritis Rheum 1997; 40: 1189.

2. Younger DS. Vasculitis of the nervous system. Curr Opin Neurol 2004; 17: 317.

3. Calabrese LH, Furlan AJ, Gragg LA, Ropos TJ. Primary angiitis of the central nervous system: diagnostic criteria and clinical approach. Cleve Clin J Med 1992; 59: 293.

4. Pomper MG, Miller TJ, Stone JH, et al. CNS vasculitis in autoimmune disease: MR imaging findings and correlation with angiography. AJNR Am J Neuroradiol 1999; 20: 75.

5. Lie JT. Classification and histopathologic spectrum of central nervous system vasculitis. Neurol Clin 1997; 15: 805.

Chapter 18

Sodium disorders

Mypinder S. Sekhon and Donald E. Griesdale

Sodium is the principle extracellular cation and an important osmotically active agent. Disorders of sodium/water balance can result in catastrophic neurological consequences through their pathophysiological consequences and inappropriate management.

Hyponatremia

- Pathophysiology.
- Usually an excess of total body water relative to sodium.
- Anti diuretic hormone (ADH) is predominantly responsible for this phenomenon. ADH can either be appropriate (hypovolemia or decreased effective circulating volume related stimuli) or inappropriate (syndrome of inappropriate ADH release – SIADH).
- Less commonly, kidneys are unable to maintain a normal serum sodium due to high urinary Na losses (cerebral salt wasting, thiazide diuretics, mineralocorticoid deficiency).

Table 18.1 Approach to hyponatremia etiology

Category	Urine studies	Etiology
Hypervolemic	$U_{Na+} > 20$ mEq/l	Renal failure
	$U_{Na+} < 10$ mEq/l	Congestive heart failure, cirrhosis, nephrotic syndrome
Euvolemic	$U_{OSM} > 100$	SIADH, hypothyroidism, glucocorticoid deficiency
	$U_{OSM} < 100$	1 polydipsia, low solute intake (*tea & toast*)
	U_{OSM} variable	Reset osmostat
Hypovolemic	$U_{Na+} > 20$ mEq/l	Renal losses (cerebral salt wasting, thiazides, mineralocorticoid deficiency
	$U_{Na+} < 10$ mEq/l	Extra renal losses (third spacing, GI/insensible losses)

Table 18.2 Differentiating cerebral salt wasting vs. SIADH by etiology

	Cerebral salt wasting (CSW)	SIADH

Causes	a. SAH
	  • Most common cause of CSW
	b. TBI
	c. Gliomas
	d. Meningitis
		a. Pulmonary
		  • Pneumonia
		  • Small cell lung cancer
		  • COPD/asthma
		b. CNS
		  • Stroke/ICH
		  • SAH/TBI
		  • Infection/tumor
		  • Hydrocephalus
		c. Drugs
		  • Anti depressants
		  • Anti-psychotics
		d. Other
		  • Pain/nausea/post op

Table 18.3 Differentiating cerebral salt wasting vs. SIADH

		Cerebral salt wasting	SIADH
Pathophysiology	Mechanisms	ANP/BNP induced naturesis	Elevated ADH and water reabsorption
	Plasma volume	Low	Normal or elevated
	Sodium balance	Negative	Neutral
	Water balance	Neutral	Positive
Clinical	Volume status	Negative	Euvolemia/hypervolemia
	Orthostatic vitals	Present	Absent
	JVP	Flat	Normal or elevated
	Skin turgor	Decreased	Normal
	Sunken eyes	Present	Absent
	Mucous membranes	Dry	Normal
	Daily weight	Decreased	Even
	Daily fluid balance	Negative	Even/positive

Table 18.3 (cont.)

		Cerebral salt wasting	SIADH
Investigations	Serum Na	Low	Low
	Serum osmolality	Normal or elevated	Low
	Urine Na	Normal or elevated	Normal or high
	Urine osmolality	Elevated	High
	Hematocrit	Elevated	Normal
	BUN/Cr	Elevated	Normal
Diagnosis		Hyponatremia with features of hypovolemia in the context of the above mentioned causes	Hyponatremia with a biochemical profile indicating high ADH and euvolemic state
Treatment		a. 0.9% normal saline b. 3–5% hypertonic saline c. Fludrocortisone	a. Free H_2O restriction b. 3–5% hypertonic saline c. Demecocycline/Li^+ d. V2 receptor antagonism
Rate of Na correction		a. Asymptomatic: 0.5 mEq/l/h b. Symptomatic: 1–2 mEq/l/h × 2–3 hours until symptoms resolve c. Maximum 10–12 mEq/l/24 hours	
Complication of rapid Na correction		Osmotic dymelination syndrome (ODS) – Occurs with rapidly corrected serum sodium in the setting of prolonged hyponatremia (> 48 h). In the setting of prolonged hyponatremia, neurons degrade intracellular organic osmoles to avoid intracellular edema when exposed to the relative hypotonic extracellular environment. If the serum sodium is then raised precipitously, the neurons do not have enough time to regenerate these organic intracellular osmoles and intracellular water can be drawn out of the intracellular compartment, resulting in widespread neuronal damage, which manifests as ODS.	

Hypernatremia

Pathophysiology

- Usually a deficit of water relative to sodium.
- Can occur from losses of hypotonic fluid from kidneys or extrarenal sources.
- Less commonly, can result from an excessive sodium load from hypertonic fluids resulting in an increased serum osmolality, which the kidneys cannot overcome via water retention.

Table 18.4 Approach to etiology of hypernatremia

Category	Urine studies	Etiology
Hypervolemic	U_{osm} 300–600 U_{Na} > 20 U_{osm} > 600 U_{Na} < 20	Renal hypotonic fluid losses Extrarenal hypotonic fluid losses
Euvolemic	U_{osm} < 300 U_{osm} 300–600	Diabetes insipidus (central or nephrogenic) Partial diabetes insipidus
Hypovolemic	None	Exogenous sodium load (hypertonic saline) Mineralocorticoid excess

Central diabetes insipidus is a state which occurs from an inability to produce or release antidiuretic hormone (ADH) from the hypothalamic–pituitary axis and leads to free water loss at the level of the nephron, ultimately resulting in hypernatremia.

Table 18.5 Pathophysiology and etiology of central diabetes insipidus

Anatomical site	Etiology
Hypothalamus	SAH TBI Meningoencephalitis ICH
Hypophyseal stalk	Malignancy Pituitary surgery
Posterior pituitary	Malignancy Ant. pit. adenoma Radiation Vasculitis Pituitary surgery Pituitary stunning post cerebral injury – triple phase response

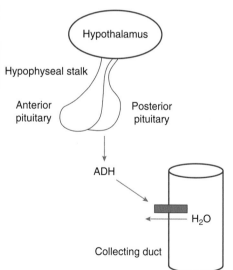

Figure 18.1 Pathophysiology and etiology of central diabetes insipidus.

Diagnosis

- Polyuria usually 3–4 l/24 h of urine output.
- Water deprivation test:
  - Usually done as an outpatient or in a non-critical setting.
  - The patient is deprived of enteral water intake while serum sodium, osmolality and urine osmolality is measured every 30 minutes to 1 hour. Continue water deprivation until serum osmolality is > 295 mosm/l and urine osmolality is < 300 mosm/l. Administer DDAVP and if the urine osmolality increases by 50%, then central DI is confirmed
- Urine and serum osmolality.
  - The urine osmolality in central DI is usually < 300 mosm/l. Obtain simultaneous urine and serum osmolalities. In the setting of hypernatremia and polyuria, if the urine osmolality is less than 300 mosm/l and less than the serum osmolality, then central DI is likely. This indicates an ADH deficient state. Upon administering DDAVP, the collecting duct should start reabsorbing water and the urine out and serum Na should correct. This confirms central DI.

Table 18.6 Management options of central diabetes insipidus

Treatment	Notes
DDAVP	Treatment of choice. Can be given intranasally, parenterally or orally. Starting dose is usually 1–2 mcg IV every 8–12 hours. Titrate to urine output and serum sodium.
Chlorpropamide	Increases the sensitivity of the ADH receptors in the collecting duct.
Carbamazepine	Increases the sensitivity of the ADH receptors in the collecting duct. Reduces the osmoregulatory threshold for ADH secretion from the posterior pituitary.
Clofibrate	Stimulates ADH production in the hypothalamus.

Summary

- Hyponatremia and hypernatremia are common metabolic derangements in the neurocritically ill patient.
- Hyponatremia is most often caused by cerebral salt wasting or SIADH in neurocritical patients after various causes of brain injury.
- Distinguishing CSW vs. SIADH requires a careful evaluation of total body volume status. It is important to make this distinction as the therapy for CSW and SIADH differs.
- Hypernatremia is most commonly caused by central diabetes insipidus in the neurocritically ill patient. Characteristically, central DI results in excretion of dilute urine in large amounts (polyuria), which can result in precipitous elevations in serum sodium. Prompt identification, evaluation and therapy involves careful assessment of serum/urine electrolyte concentrations and osmolality. DDAVP is the mainstay of treatment.

Suggested readings

1. Bradshaw K, Smith M. Disorders of sodium balance after brain injury. BJA. 2008;8(4):129–133.

2. Rabinstein AA, Wijdicks EF. Hyponatremia in critically ill neurological patients. Neurologist. 2003;9:290–300.

3. Wright WL. Sodium and fluid management in acute brain injury. Curr Neurol Neurosci Rep. 2012;12(4):466–473.

4. Diringer MN, Zazulia AR. Hyponatremia in neurologic patients: consequences and approaches to treatment. Neurologist. 2006;12(3):117–126.

5. Nathan BR. Cerebral correlates of hyponatremia. Neurocrit Care. 2007;6(1):72–78

Chapter 19

Paroxysmal sympathetic hyperactivity

Mypinder S. Sekhon and
Donald E. Griesdale

Definition: Paroxysmal sympathetic hyperactivity (PSH) is a clinical entity frequently encountered in neurocritically ill patients, which exhibits manifestations of excessive sympathetic output and catecholamine discharges resulting in end-organ dysfunction from hyperthermia, diaphoresis, tachycardia, hypertension, tachypnea and dystonic posturing.

Table 19.1 Etiology of paroxysmal sympathetic hyperactivity

Cause	Percentage (%)
Traumatic brain injury	60–70
Subarachnoid hemorrhage	7–10
Anoxic brain injury	5–7
Intracranial hemorrhage	5
Encephalitis	5
Ischemic stroke	2
Thalamic tumor	2
Vasculitis	1
Multiple sclerosis	1

Table 19.2 Risk factors for paroxysmal sympathetic hyperactivity

Category		Notes
Demographic	Age	Young age, predominantly < 40
	Sex	Higher male predominance. Biased by increased males suffering TBI
Clinical	Injury	Traumatic brain injury
	Grade of injury	Greatly increased risk of severe grade (GCS < 8)
	Timing	Episodes occur 5–7 days post injury. Usually during weaning of sedative agents
Imaging	Location of injury	Deep nuclei, corpus callosum, brainstem
	Type of injury	Diffuse axonal injury Associated epidural or subdural hematoma

Pathophysiology

- Functional disconnection or unbalanced sympathetic nervous system activation, beyond the ability to maintain autonomic control.
- Excitatory–inhibitory model: Autonomic efferent activity at the level of the spinal cord is mediated by inhibitory inputs from the diencephalon or mesencephalon. After brain injury, the constant inhibitory inputs from the cortex and brainstem are disrupted, resulting in unopposed sympathetic efferent output. This results in the imbalance of peripheral adrenergic outflow and end-organ effects. Thereafter, there is a positive feedback loop whereby any stimuli (non-noxious) results in an excessive adrenergic response.

Diagnosis

Although there are no accepted universal diagnostic criteria currently, a few have been proposed in the literature.

Proposed diagnostic criteria (Mayo Clinic):

- Rule out alternative mimicking diagnoses:
  - Sepsis
  - Substance withdrawal
  - Opiate or benzodiazepine withdrawal
  - Serotonin syndrome
  - Neuroleptic malignant syndrome
  - New or worsening brain injury

Table 19.3 Clinical manifestations of paroxysmal sympathetic hyperactivity

Sign/symptom	Frequency (%)
Tachycardia	98
Tachypnea	85
Fever	80
Diaphoresis	75
Hypertension	70
Dystonia	40
Posturing	40

- More than one episode of at least four of:
  - Fever (temperature > 38.3°C)
  - Tachycardia (heart rate > 120 beats/min or > 100 beats/min if on beta blocker)
  - Hypertension (BP > 160 mmHg or > 140 mmHg if on beta blocker)
  - Tachypnea (respiratory rate > 25 breaths/min)
  - Diaphoresis
  - Presence of dystonic posturing
  - Rigidity or spasticity

Treatment

General approach

- Confirm diagnosis by excluding other mimicking conditions such as sepsis, opiate/benzodiazepine withdrawal, agitation, delirium, serotonin syndrome and neuroleptic malignant syndrome.
- Initiate regularly dosed standing medications to decrease frequency and intensity of episodes. Abortive medications with short-acting properties should be used to terminate paroxysms if they occur as breakthrough.

Table 19.4 Management of paroxysmal sympathetic hyperactivity

Treatment	Mechanism of action/notes
Clonidine	Presynaptic alpha 2 agonist. Reduces sympathetic outflow from hypothalamus and medulla.
Dexmedetomidine	Intravenous alpha 2 agonist. Similar to clonidine in that it reduces sympathetic outflow.
Gabapentin	Analog of GABA. Titrate dose to 300–600 mg every 8 hours. Case series have suggested benefit in PSH.
Baclofen	GABA analog and GABA^B agonist. Intrathecal baclofen reported beneficial in PSH. However, conventional therapies should be attempted initially.
Beta blockers	Diminish peripheral effects of catecholamines. Diaphoresis, dystonic posturing have also been reported to respond to beta blockers. Propanolol (non-selective) is the agent of choice.
Benzodiazepines	GABA receptor agonists. Use as short-acting abortive medications for breakthrough paroxysms.
Bromocriptine	Synthetic dopamine agonist. Stimulates D2 receptors and antagonizes D1 receptors in hypothalamus/striatium. Case reports of possible benefits if used with other agents for PSH.
Morphine	Potent mu receptor agonist. Stimulates medullary vagal nuclei resulting in cholinergic effects.
Dantrolene	Use if dystonia or posturing is refractory to all other therapies. Caution with concurrent liver impairment/disease.

Summary

- Paroxysmal sympathetic hyper-reflexia is a complex condition resulting from periodic catecholamine-induced surges which manifest as symptoms/signs of catecholamine excess and neurological abnormalities.
- The most common etiology of PSH is TBI, followed by SAH, anoxic brain injury, ICH, encephalitis and stroke.

- There are currently no consensus diagnostic criteria; however, mimicking conditions such as sepsis, opiate/benzodiazepine withdrawal and toxicology syndromes must be excluded prior to establishing a firm diagnosis of PSH.
- Management involves the use of multiple pharmacological approaches including GABA agonists, beta blockers, sympatholytics, dopamine agonists and muscle relaxants.

Suggested readings

1. Choi AC, Jeon SB, Samuel S, Allison T, Lee K. Paroxysmal sympathetic hyperactivity after acute brain injury. Curr Neurol Neurosci Rep. 2013. 13: 370–376.

2. Hughes JD, Rabinstein AA. Early diagnosis of paroxysmal sympathetic hyperactivity in the ICU. Neurocrit Care. 2013. 13:987–983.

3. Perkes I, Baguley IJ, Nott MT, Menon DK. A review of paroxysmal sympathetic hyperactivity after acquired brain injury. Ann Neurol. 2010. 60:126–135.

Neurological complications of systemic disorders

Mypinder S. Sekhon and
Donald E. Griesdale

Table 20.1 Septic encephalopathy

Definition	Cerebral dysfunction occuring in the setting of sepsis
Pathogenesis	Inflammatory cascades/toxins from microbes can lead to abnormal endothelial function, neuronal metabolism, mitochondrial dysfunction, abnormal signaling and free radical injury. Sepsis can also result in systemic metabolic abnormalities such as hepatic/renal dysfunction and electrolytes disorders, which may cause abnormal neuronal function.
Manifestations	Altered LOC, confusion, stupor, delirium
Diagnosis	Evidence of central nervous system dysfunction (RASS Scale) in the setting of sepsis while excluding potential confounders.
Treatment	Treat underlying source of sepsis Correct metabolic derangements Manage delirium, if present Minimize sedation, if possible

Table 20.2 Cerebral edema in setting of fulminant hepatic failure

Definition	Cerebral edema occuring in the setting of fulminant hepatic failure
Etiology	Can occur secondary to any etiology that results in fulminant hepatic failure; 80% of patient deaths from fulminant hepatic failure are secondary to cerebral herniation from uncontrolled cerebral edema.

Table 20.2 (cont.)

Pathogenesis	Cytotoxic edema occurs secondary to an accumulation of intracellular glutamate from elevated systemic ammonia, which acts as an intracellular osmole, thereby drawing water into the intracellular compartment. Inflammatory cascades cause a disruption of the blood–brain barrier. Coupled with a characteristic hyperemic state, vasogenic edema can ensue.
Manifestations	Altered LOC, upper motor neuron signs Signs of increased ICP – Cushing's reflex (bradycardia and hypertension) Herniation
Diagnosis	Altered LOC with evidence of cerebral edema or increased ICP (radiographic of clinical) in the setting of fulminant hepatic failure.
Treatment	ICP monitoring is level IIb recommendation. Risks of intracranial bleeding are increased because of concurrent coagulopathy. Empirical treatment: a. Maintain sedation (ideally with short-acting agents – propofol but concurrent hemodynamic disturbances may prohibit its judicial use) b. Osmotherapy – hypertonic saline, mannitol c. Normothermia to mild hypothermia (35–36°C) d. Normocapnia (PaCO$_2$ 35–40 mmHg) e. Head of bed elevation 30 degrees, ensure ETT tie not restricting jugular vein flow Neck in neutral position f. Evaluate for concurrent non-convulsive seizures – obtain EEG

Table 20.3 Hepatic encephalopathy

Definition	Encephalopathy resulting in the setting of concurrent cirrhosis
Precipitants	Infection – sepsis, spontaneous bacterial peritonitis Upper GI bleed Constipation Electrolyte disturbances – hypokalemia, metabolic alkalosis, volume depletion Meds – sedative agents (benzodiazepines), psychoactive medications Portosystemic shunt Renal failure
Pathogenesis	Ammonia accumulation causing neuronal dysfunction
Manifestations	Stage 1 – Day night reversal Stage 2 – Asterixis present Stage 3 – Confusion, stupor, upper motor neuron signs Stage 4 – Coma, decerebrate posturing

Table 20.3 (cont.)

Diagnosis	Clinical diagnosis
Treatment	Correct underlying precipitant Lactulose – acidification of stool leading to trapping of NH_4^+ within colon lumen. Titrate to 3–4 stools per day Gut decontamination with rifamixin or neomycin may have benefit by decreasing NH_3 producing organisms. Not routinely used currently

Table 20.4 Uremic encephalopathy

Definition	Encephalopathy which occurs in the setting of either acute or acute on chronic renal failure.
Etiology	Any cause of acute renal failure that produces significant increases in urea
Pathogenesis	Accumulation of nephrotoxins leads to altered neuronal metabolism, functioning and signaling.
Manifestations	Altered LOC, confusion, stupor Asterixis Seizures, status epilepticus in severe cases
Diagnosis	Encephalopathy occuring in the setting of extreme rises in urea without other possible confounder.
Treatment	Treat underlying cause for renal failure, if possible Hemodialysis

Dialysis dysequilibrium	
Definition	Cerebral edema resulting from precipitous decrease in serum urea concentrations.
Pathogenesis	With chronic elevations in urea, neurons adapt by creating intracellular osmoles such as taurine, phosphocreatinine, myoinosotal, gulatamate. During initial hemodialysis, if urea decreases rapidly, the intracellular osmoles cause water shift into the intracellular compartment and result in cerebral edema.
Manifestations	Altered LOC, upper motor signs, headache, nausea Signs of increased ICP Cerebral edema
Prevention	Short initial run of hemodialysis Ramp sodium concentrations in dialysate Use low flow rate for initial run
Treatment	Use osmotically active agents (hypertonic saline) to increase serum osmolality to decrease cerebral edema.

Table 20.5 Hypertensive encephalopathy

Definition	The presence of cerebral edema caused by breakthrough hyperperfusion from severe hypertension.
Etiology	Any cause of malignant hypertension.
Pathogenesis	Severe hypertension results in autoregulation failure, and breakthrough vasodilation causes cerebral edema. With extreme hypertension, the cerebral vascular endothelium becomes dysfunctional and the tight blood–brain barrier can become compromised, thereby leading to vasogenic edema.
Manifestations	Altered LOC, upper motor neuron signs Cerebral edema can lead to increased ICP and herniation in extreme cases
Imaging	Evidence of cerebral edema (sulcal effacement, basal cistern effacement, herniation, lateral ventricle collapse).
Diagnosis	Clinical diagnosis
Treatment	Decrease mean arterial pressure by ~ 25% with 2 h using intravenous agents Agents: labetolol, nitroglycerin, nitroprusside, hydralazine

Table 20.6 Posterior reversible encephalopathy syndrome

Definition	Clinical entity characterized by cerebral edema in vascular supply of the posterior circulation accompanied by radiographic evidence of cerebral edema in this location.
Etiology	HELLP syndrome Pre-eclampsia Medications – mycophenylate, tacrolimus, sirolimus, oxaliplatin, bevacizumab, gemcitabine, cyclosporine
Pathogenesis	The posterior circulation is relatively devoid of sympathetic input. In states of extreme systemic hypertension, breakthrough vasodilation results in the posterior circulation and leads to vasogenic cerebral edema.
Manifestations	Headache, altered LOC, cortical vision impairment
Imaging	Isolated cerebral edema in the distribution of the vascular supply of the posterior circulation. Predominantly occipital lobe involvement.

Table 20.6 (cont.)

Diagnosis	Clinical risk factors, presentation and characteristic radiographic characteristics.
Treatment	Treat underlying predisposing condition Decrease MAP ~ 25% with intravenous agents Remove potential offending medications

Table 20.7 Neurological manifestations of bacterial endocarditis

Ischemic stroke	Most common CNS complication: bacterial endocarditis Embolic phenomenon from detached vegetation Vegetations > 1 cm have higher risk of embolization If cerebral ischemic stroke occurs with right-sided endocarditis, then evaluate for right to left intracardiac shunt or intrapulmonary shunt/AVM
Mycotic aneurysms	Microembolization to cerebral vasculature results in intraluminal infection. Subsequent intima/media/adventitial weakening leading to aneurysm formation.
Intracranial hemorrhage	Can occur from mycotic aneurysm rupture. Subarachnoid and intracerebral hemorrhage are most common. Intracerebral hemorrhage usually occurs from hemorrhagic transformation of ischemic strok.
Intracranial abscess	Microembolization leads to subclinical ischemic stroke. Subsequent impairment of the blood–brain barrier in this region makes the cerebral parenchyma susceptible to bacterial invasion, infection and abscess formation.
Seizures	Can result secondary to ischemic stroke, intracranial hemorrhage or abscess.

Table 20.8 Paraneoplastic associated neurological dysfunction

Pathology	Associated malignancy
Cerebellar degeneration	Loss of cerebellar Purkinje cells Associated with small cell lung or ovarian cancer
Opsoclonus–myoclonus	Involuntary, arrhythmic, multidirectional, high-amplitude conjugate saccades Associated with neuroblastoma

Table 20.8 (cont.)

Pathology		Associated malignancy
Encephalitis	Limbic encephalitis	Ovarian, lung, neuroblastoma, testicular, breast, thymus, thyroid, renal, uterine
	Rhomboencephalitis	Ovarian, breast, lung
	Diencephalitis	Lung, neuroblastoma, breast, testicular
	Cerebellar encephalitis	Lung, thymus, ovarian, breast, uterine
Peripheral neuropathy		Anti-Hu antibody associated neuropathy. Occurs with small cell lung cancer
Lambert–Eaton		Antibody against presynaptic voltage-gated calcium channel receptor Occurs with small cell lung cancer
Myasthenia gravis		Common association with thymoma

Table 20.9 Neurological manifestations of endocrine disease

Thyroid storm	Anxiety, tremulousness, tremor, psychosis Altered LOC Extreme hyperthermia leading to seizures in extreme cases Ischemic stroke (from atrial fibrillation associated with hyperthyroidism)
Myxedema coma	Altered LOC Hypoglycemia can lead to neuroglycopenia and onset of seizures Hyponatremia in severe cases causing altered LOC
Hashimoto's encephalitis	Autoimmune condition associated with Hashimoto's thyroiditis Presents gradually over 3–7 days with symptoms: a. Movement disorders (tremors, myoclonus, ataxia) b. Psychiatric symptoms (depression, anxiety, psychosis, delusions, coma, attention difficulties, personality changes) c. Focal neurological symptoms (aphasia, focal deficit) d. Seizures, status epilepticus
Cushing's syndrome	Depression, psychosis, anxiety Myopathy (proximal muscle groups predominantly)
DKA/HONK	Altered LOC results from associated electrolyte disturbances or acidemia (DKA). Precipitants of DKA/HONK, such as sepsis or cerebral vascular ischemic events, can also primarily account for altered LOC.

Table 20.10 Neurological manifestations of nutritional defiencies

Vitamin	Neurological complication
Thiamine (B1)	Coenzyme for decarboxylation of α-keto acids, and acts as a cofactor for transketolase. Deficiency of thiamine results in reduced oxygen uptake and lactic acid accumulation in CNS tissues. Leads to Wernicke's encephalopathy and Korsakoff's syndrome. Also can lead to peripheral neuropathy and cortical cerebellar degeneration.
Pyridoxine (B6)	Deficiency results in distal symmetric polyneuropathy
Cobalamin (B12)	Deficiency can lead to dementia-like syndromes and posterior column spinal cord degeneration. Also associated with peripheral polyneuropathy.
Nicotonic acid	Psychiatric manifestations: depression, mania, confusion, memory impairment Extrapyramidal or cerebellar manifestations can occur
Vitamin E	Deficiency can result in spinocerebellar degeneration and polyneuropathy.

Table 20.11 Critical care polyneuropathy

Definition	Polyneuropathy which occurs in the setting of critical illness and with other etiologies ruled out.
Risk factors	Sepsis, shock, vasopressors, prolonged mechanical ventilation, multiorgan failure, renal failure, total parenteral nutrition, hyperglycemia. Intravenous sedation, neuromuscluar paralysis, glucocorticoid use, immobilization.
Pathogenesis	Multiple insults (metabolic, bioenergetic, inflammatory alterations) lead to gradual denervation of peripheral nerves, leading to a symmetric peripheral axonal neuropathy.
Diagnosis	a. Presence of sepsis, multiorgan failure, respiratory failure, SIRS b. Difficulty weaning from ventilator or symmetric limb weakness c. Decreased amplitudes on electromyography d. Widespread denervation potentials in muscle e. Normal CK, rule out other causes of peripheral neuropathy
Treatment	Stop all potential offending pharamcological agents Treat underlying condition Wean off mechanical ventilation, if possible Mobilization and physiotherapy

Summary

- Systemic conditions such as sepsis, acute and chronic liver disease, acute kidney injury, uremia, hypertensive disorders, nutritonal deficiencies and endocrinopathies can result in nervous system manifestations.
- Critical care neuropathy results from the denervation of myelinated axons and is associated with worse outcomes.
- Management of CNS manifestations of systemic diseases requires reversal of the underlying condition and simultaneous consideration of neurospecific therapies to reverse underlying pathophysiology (i.e., lactulose in hepatic encephalopathy).

Suggested readings

1. Papadopoulos MC, Davies DC, Moss RF, Tighe D, Bennett ED. Pathophysiology of septic enecephalopathy: a review. Crit Care Med. 2000. 28(8):3019–3024.

2. Dbouk N, McGuire BM. Hepatic encephaloptahy: a review of its pathophysiology and treatment. Curr Treat Options Gastroenterol. 2006. 9(6):464–474.

3. Hermans G, De Jonghe B, Bruyninckx, Van den Burghe G. Clinical review: Critical illness polyneuropathy and myopathy. Crit Care. 2008. 12(6):238.

4. Schwartz RB. Hyperperfusion encephalopathies: hypertensive encephalopathy and related conditions. Neurologist. 2002. 8(1):22–34.

5. Seifter JL, Samuels MA. Uremic encephalopathy and other brain disorders associated with renal failure. Semin Neurol. 2001. 31(20):139–143.

Central nervous system toxicology

Mypinder S. Sekhon and
William R. Henderson

Table 21.1 Common toxidromes and associated clinical signs

Toxidrome	Signs	
Benzodiazepine	a. Depressed level of conciousness b. Bradypnea/apnea	
Opioid	a. Depressed level of conciousness b. Bradypnea/apnea c. Miosis	
Sympathomimetic	a. Tachycardia b. Hypertension c. Hyperthermia d. Tachypnea	e. Diaphoresis f. Mydriasis g. Flushing
Anticholinergic	a. Tachycardia b. Mydriasis c. Hyperthermia d. Flushing	e. Dry skin/mucous membranes f. Urinary retention g. Absent bowel sounds
Cholinergic	a. Bradycardia b. Lacrimation c. Urinary/fecal incontinence d. Salivation	
Serotonin syndrome	a. Hyperthermia b. Autonomic instability c. Rigidity d. Mental status altered e. Hyper-reflexia (LE > UE) f. Clonus	
NMS	a. Hyperthermia b. Autonomic instability c. Rigidity d. Mental status altered	

Table 21.2 Suggested investigations for suspected poisoning

Investigation	Purpose
Complete blood count	Leukocytosis common with Li^+ overdose
Electrolytes	Calculation of anion gap
Arterial blood gas	Determining acid–base balance for specific poisonings
Urinalysis/screen	Detects benzodiazepines/opiates/cocaine/amphetamines
Liver enzymes	Determination of underlying liver disease – may effect metabolism of certain poisonings
Electrocardiogram	QRS and R wave morphology in context of tricyclic antidepressant overdose Evaluation of QTc in context of antidepressant overdose – risk of torsades de pointes
Serum levels	Salicylate Acetaminophen Li^+
Radiography a. Chest X-ray b. Abdominal X-ray	Evaluate for acute respiratory distress syndrome/aspiration (if decreased LOC) Iron can be visualized after ingestion

Table 21.3 Diagnosis and management of benzodiazepine overdose

Benzodiazepine overdose	
Culprit drugs	All benzodiazepine class medications – predominantly exert effects via GABA receptor inhibition
Clinical manifestations	Classic toxidrome – depressed level of conciousness and respiratory rate with normal cardiovascular/autonomic nervous system signs

Treatment	a. Discontinuation of all precipitating agents
	b. Supportive care
	  – Airway support
	  – Mechanical ventilation if indication for intubation
	c. Antagonists
	  – Flumazenil – use caution if coingestions as may precipitate refractory seizures

Table 21.4 Diagnosis and management of opioid overdose

Opioid overdose	
Culprit drugs	All opiate receptor agonists a. Morphine d. Hydromorphone b. Codeine e. Remifentanil c. Fentanyl f. Oxycodone
Clinical manifestations	a. Decreased level of consciousness b. Miosis c. Bradypnea/apnea

Treatment	a. Discontinuation of all precipitating agents
	b. Supportive care
	  – Airway support
	  – Mechanical ventilation if indication for intubation
	c. Antagonists
	  – Naloxone – 0.1 to 0.4mg IV. Consider infusion if sustained release product. Caution to avoid hyperalgesia with bolus dose of naloxone > 0.4 mg

Table 21.5 Diagnosis and management of sympathomimetic overdose

Sympathomimetic overdose	
Culprit drugs	Cocaine Methamphetamines Ecstasy Methylphenidate Ephedrine/pseudoephedrine
Clinical manifestations	a. Sympathomimetic toxidrome b. Seizures c. Acute respiratory distress syndrome d. Myocardial ischemia/infarction/cardiac arrest e. Rhabdomyolysis f. Disseminated intravcasular coagulation
Treatment	a. Discontinuation of all precipitating agents b. Supportive care c. Benzodiazepine sedation d. Control of fever/hyperthermia

Table 21.6 Diagnosis and management of tricyclic antidepressant overdose

Tricyclic antidepressant overdose	
Culprit drugs	Amitryptyline Nortryptyline
Clinical manifestations	a. Toxidrome – anticholinergic b. Results in Na^+ blockade c. QRS > 120 msec = increased risk of seizures d. QRS > 160 msec = increased risk of VT/VF e. Terminal R wave in aVR = increased risk of VT/VF f. Alpha blockade in peripheral vasculature and catecholamine release inhibition results in cardiac collapse
Treatment	a. Discontinuation of all precipitating agents b. Sodium bicarbonate – to overcome Na^+ blockade – if pH > 7.55, then hypertonic saline to overcome TCA induced Na^+ blockade c. Norephinephrine/epinephrine infusion in setting of cardiovascular collapse (to overcome alpha receptor blockade) d. If seizures, avoid phenytoin administration because of additional Na^+ blockade

Table 21.7 Diagnosis and management of salicylate overdose

Salicylate overdose	
Culprit drugs	Acetylsalicylic acid
Clinical manifestations	a. Decreased level of conciousness/seizures secondary to neuroglycopenia b. Uncouples oxidative phosphorylation at mitochondria c. Anion gap metabolic acidosis secondary to lactate d. Medullary stimulation resulting in respiratory alkalosis e. Acute respiratory distress syndrome

Treatment	a. Discontinuation of all precipitating agents
	b. Ion trapping – $NaHCO_3$ to promote dissociation of salicylate anion and prevent reabsorption in renal tubules/diffusion into brain parenchyma
	c. Dialysis if:
	   – pH < 7.2
	   – Lactate > 4
	   – Salicylate level > 6.0
	   – Signs of end-organ dysfunction (CNS/pulmonary)
	d. Supportive care
	   – Airway support
	   – Mechanical ventilation if depressed LOC or ARDS

Table 21.8 Diagnosis and management of serotonin syndrome

Serotonin syndrome	
Culprit drugs	Increased serotonin intake a. Tryptophan Decreased serotonin breakdown a. Linezolid b. Ritonavir c. MAOIs Increased serotonin release a. Sympathomimetics – cocaine, amphetamines Decreased serotonin reuptake a. SSRIs b. Dextromethorphan c. Merperidine d. Tramadol e. Fentanyl Serotonin receptor agonists a. Triptans b. Lithium
Clinical manifestations	Fever – > 40°C in extreme cases Autonomic instability – Tachycardia, hypertension, diaphoresis, increased enteric motility Neuromuscular rigidity, clonus, hyper-reflexia – Typically greater in lower extremities Mental status change

Diagnosis	Clinical
	Hunter's criteria
	a. History of serotonergic agent intake
	b. One of the following
	    – Spontaneous clonus
	    – Inducible clonus + agitation or diaphoresis
	    – Tremor and hyper-reflexia
	    – Hypertonia
	    – Temp > 38°C + ocular clonus

Treatment	a. Discontinuation of all serotonergic agents
	b. Benzodiazepine sedation
	c. Supportive care
	    – Intravenous fluid administration
	    – Blood pressure control (clonidine if HTN)
	    – Cooling to achieve normothermia
	d. Non-depolarizing neuromuscular blockade
	    – If continued rigidity and hyperthermia resistant to
	      above mentioned therapies. Ensure endotracheal intubation
	e. Serotonergic antagonists
	    – Cyproheptadine – 5-HT1A and 5-HT2A antagonist
	      12 mg enteric load, then 6–8mg every 6 hours

Table 21.9 Diagnosis and management of neuroleptic malignant syndrome

Neuroleptic malignant syndrome	
Culprit drugs	Anti-psychotics a. Typicals – haloperidol, clozapine, fluphenazine b. Atypicals – olanzapine, respiridone, quetiapine Anti-emetics a. Metoclopramide b. Prochlorperazine c. Promethazine
Clinical manifestations	Fever Autonomic instability Neuromuscular rigidity Mental status change

Diagnosis	DSM-IV criteria
	a. Development of severe rigidity and elevated temperature associated with the use of neuroleptic medication
	b. Two of the following:
	  – Diaphoresis – Dysphagia
	  – Tremor – Incontinence
	  – Change LOC – Mutism
	  – Tachycardia – Elevated or labile BP
	  – Leukocytosis – Elevated CK
	
	c. Not due to another substance, or neurological Dx or other general medical condition

Treatment	a. Remove offending agent
	b. Benzodiazepines
	  – Lorazepam or midazolam–ensure adequate airway control
	c. Bromocriptine–2.5mg q8h, increase to 10 mg q8h
	d. Dantrolene–1 to 2.5mg/kg IV × 1 then 1mg/kg IV q6h
	e. Supportive therapy
	  – Intravenous fluid administration
	  – Blood pressure control (clonidine if HTN)
	  – Cooling to achieve normothermia
	f. Non-depolarizing neuromuscular blockade
	  – If continued rigidity and hyperthermia resistant to above mentioned therapies. Ensure endotracheal intubation

Table 21.10 Diagnosis and management of organophosphate poisoning

Organophosphate poisoning

Culprit drugs	Insecticides (malathion, parathion, diazinon, fenthion)
	Nerve gases (Sarin)
	Ophthalmic agents (echothiophate, isoflurophate)
	Antihelmintics (trichlorfon)
	Herbicides (tribufos)
Clinical manifestations	Muscarinic cholinergic effects:
	Salivation
	Lacrimation
	Urination
	Diarrhea
	GI upset
	Emesis
Diagnosis	Clinical diagnosis with exposure history
Treatment	A–Airway protection (excess secretions require endotracheal intubation)
	B–Difficulty with ventilation due to bronchospasm and airway secretions. Require aggressive bronchial suctuoning and bronchodilators
	C–Bradycardia with cardiovascular collapse. Atropine used to reverse cholinergic effects on chonotropy. Other treatments– pralidoxime. If seizures then treatment with intravenous benzodiazepines (midazolam)

Table 21.11 Diagnosis and management of malignant hyperthermia

Malignant Hyperthermia

Culprit drugs	Halogenated inhaled anesthetics
	– Halothane, isoflurane, sevoflurane, desflurane, enflurane
	Succinylcholine
Clinical manifestations	a. Muscle rigidity
	b. Increased end tidal CO_2
	c. Hyperthermia (especially > 40°C)
	d. Elevated serum creatinine kinase–rhabdomyolysis
	e. Tachycardia & tachypnea

Table 21.11 (cont.)

Malignant Hyperthermia

Treatment	a. Discontinuation of all precipitating agents
	b. Supportive care
	   – Intravenous fluid administration
	   – Cooling to achieve normothermia
	   – Tx electrolyte disorders–especially hyperkalemia
	   – 100% FiO_2
	c. Dantrolene–1 to 2.5mg/kg IV × 1 then 1mg/kg IV q6h

Table 21.12 Diagnosis and management of toxic alcohols poisoning

Methanol overdose

Culprit drugs	Methanol
Clinical manifestations	Retinal toxicity–vision loss (formic acid induced) Anion gap metabolic acidosis Altered mental status (with profound acidemia)
Treatment	Airway, Breathing, Circulation Antidote–Fomepizole 15mg/kg loading dose. 10mg/kg IV q12h or 10mg/kg q4h during hemodialysis. Most effective if osmolar gap still elevated, indicating large amount of parent compound. Blocks alcohol dehydrogenase and prevents formation of toxic metabolites (oxalic acid) Antidote–Ethanol infusion. Limited utility with emergence of fomepizole now Elimination–Hemodialysis Folate 50mg IV every 6 hours. Promotes metabolism of parent compound to non-toxic metabolites

Ethylene Glycol overdose

Culprit drugs	Ethylene glycol
Clinical manifestations	Altered mental status (with profound acidemia) Cardiovascular collapse Anion gap metabolic acidosis Renal failure Spurious lactate elevation arterial blood gas (metabolite glycolic acid is interpreted as lactate on ABG analysis but not laboratory samples)

Table 21.12 (cont.)

Ethylene Glycol overdose	
Treatment	Airway, Breathing, Circulation
	Antidote–Fomepizole 15mg/kg loading dose. 10mg/kg IV q12h or 10mg/kg q4h during hemodialysis. Most effective if osmolar gap still elevated, indicating large amount of parent compound. Blocks alcohol dehydrogenase and prevents formation of toxic metabolites (oxalic acid)
	Antidote–Ethanol infusion. Limited utility with emergence of fomepizole now
	Elimination–Hemodialysis
	Thiamine 100mg IV every 6 hours. Promotes metabolism of parent compound to non-toxic metabolites
	Pyridoxine 25mg/kg IV every 6 hours. Promotes metabolism of parent compound to non-toxic metabolites

Table 21.13 Diagnosis and management of lithium overdose

Lithium overdose	
Culprit drugs	Lithium
Clinical manifestations	a. Decreased LOC
	b. Associated with serotonin syndrome if concomitant serotonergic agent ingestion
	c. Nephrogenic diabetes insipidus
	d. Can precipitate myxedema coma if underlying hypothyroid
	e. Low anion gap (due to elevated unmeasured Li^+ cation)
Treatment	a. Discontinuation of all precipitating agents
	b. Intravenous fluid resuscitation to promote renal clearance
	c. Management of hypernatremia in setting of nephrogenic DI
	d. Dialysis:
	– Signs of end-organ dysfunction (CNS)
	– Serum $Li^+ > 4$
	e. Supportive care

Summary

- Neuroleptic malignant syndrome, serotonin syndrome and malignant hyperthermia are three devastating toxicologic syndromes that can occur in a neurointensive care unit setting, with significant central nervous system sequelae.

- Each condition results in fever, autonomic instability and skeletal muscle damage. Neurological dysfunction is associated with extreme pyrexia, resulting in increased cerebral metabolic demand and potential permanent neuronal damage.
- Distinguishing between each diagnosis can be difficult clinically but a thorough history of culprit medications is essential.
- Management involves removal of the offending agent, antidotes and supportive therapy.

Suggested readings

1. Strawn JR, Keck PE Jr, Caroff SN. Neuroleptic malignant syndrome. Am J Psychiatry 2007; 164:870.

2. Adnet P, Lestavel P, Krivosic-Horber R. Neuroleptic malignant syndrome. Br J Anaesth 2000; 85:129.

3. Boyer EW, Shannon M. The serotonin syndrome. N Engl J Med 2005; 352:1112.

4. Lappin RI, Auchincloss EL. Treatment of the serotonin syndrome with cyproheptadine. N Engl J Med 1994; 331:1021.

5. Bodner RA, Lynch T, Lewis L, Kahn D. Serotonin syndrome. Neurology 1995; 45:219.

6. Denborough M. Malignant hyperthermia. Lancet 1998; 352:1131.

7. MacLennan DH, Phillips MS. Malignant hyperthermia. Science 1992; 256:789.

Index